D1447509

THE FUNCTIONING OF PAIRED ORGANS

K. S. ABULADZE

THE FUNCTIONING OF
PAIRED ORGANS

TRANSLATED BY

DR. R. CRAWFORD

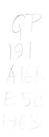

A Pergamon Press Book

THE MACMILLAN COMPANY

NEW YORK

1963

THE MACMILLAN COMPANY
60 Fifth Avenue
New York 11, N.Y.

This book is distributed by

THE MACMILLAN COMPANY · NEW YORK

pursuant to a special agreement with

PERGAMON PRESS LIMITED

Oxford, England

This translation has been made from K. S.
Abuladze's book entitled *K. voprosu o funktsii
parnykh organov*, published in Leningrad, 1961,
by Medgiz.

Library of Congress Card No. 62–22102

Printed in Great Britain by The Ditchling Press, Ditchling, Hassocks, Sussex

CONTENTS

PREFATORY NOTE

THIS book is intended for physiologists and neuropathologists. It describes some fresh material on the paired functioning of the hemispheres, obtained experimentally by means of an original method elaborated by the author. It is shown that the reflex arc for the unconditioned reflex runs on one side of the central nervous system. The reflex arc for the conditioned reflex may be situated in one or both hemispheres, depending on the methods employed for its formation. The monograph is of considerable importance for an understanding of the mechanisms of higher nervous activity.

PREFACE

THIS monograph describes some new findings on the functioning of certain paired organs and the cerebral cortex in the dog.

We have created a number of new experimental arrangements and new forms of surgical operations on dogs for the carrying out of the experiments. The surgical techniques employed by us for operation on the brain are not new in principle, but the usual methods had to be modified in detail to ensure the reliability of the special experiments we carried out in order to find an answer to our problem. As the principles of these operations have been described repeatedly by earlier authors, our review of the literature is reduced to a minimum and, in our exposition of the subject, we refer only to those findings which have a direct bearing on the various points discussed in our monograph. While we do not claim that the positions developed in our paper are absolutely correct and recognize that they may have to be modified in future, we are nevertheless convinced that the strictly objective investigation by simple yet clearly evident methods (recording of salivary secretion) helps us to advance (even if only a little) towards the truth.

K. S. ABULADZE

Leningrad.

INTRODUCTION

THE reasons for the development of paired organs, identical in anatomical structure, and the importance of bilateral symmetry for animals are obscure. All that we know is that this symmetry is first seen at the higher levels in the zoological scale and that it is steadfastly maintained in the course of further evolution, right up to man. The human organism is constructed on the principle of bilateral symmetry. It consists, as it were, of two anatomically identical, interconnected halves.

Experimental evidence and even simple everyday observations on certain paired organs make it clear that they have identical functions. The bilateral symmetry is thus functional as well as anatomical. It is also known that, when one limb is flexed, the symmetrical limb may at the same time remain at rest or may also be flexed, but to a lesser extent. So far, however, the factors determining differences in intensity or character in the simultaneous functioning of symmetrical organs have not been adequately investigated.

We started the study of this problem in experiments on paired secretory glands—salivary and lachrymal. The experiments on these glands, like other experiments which will be carried out in future, require preliminary surgical preparation of the experimental animals and the employment of special arrangements for prolonged observation on the animals, which in our case are dogs.

We shall first describe all the methods designed for this work and then discuss the experimental part of the work.

CHAPTER ONE

DESCRIPTION OF THE OPERATIONS ON DOGS AND SPECIAL ARRANGEMENTS REQUIRED FOR THE EXPERIMENTS

The Use of Ether Anaesthesia in Operations on Dogs

THE method hitherto used for the administration of ether in physiological operations is a tedious procedure, inconvenient for the anaesthetist and interfering with the surgeon. During an operation the anaesthetist usually holds the mask over the dog's muzzle with his hands. In order to pour in some more ether he raises the edge of the sterile sheet from the side of the dog's head, then raises its head and removes the mask, gets hold of the bottle containing the ether and opens it, pours ether into the mask, applies it to the dog's muzzle and then returns the dog's head and the edge of the sheet to their former positions, closes the bottle and places it on the table or in his coat pocket. During the time occupied by this procedure, the surgeon and his assistant must stop work, particularly if the operation is on or in proximity to the animal's head. All this is repeated at short intervals every time more ether has to be given.

This forced interruption of the operation is undesirable, as time is lost and work is often rendered futile as, for example, when the surgeon, finally having reached the desired part after prolonged search in the depth of the brain tissue, suddenly loses it again as a result of displacement of the dog's head in connection with the administration of a further lot of ether.

The method now used for the induction of anaesthesia also has many other defects. Correct depth of anaesthesia is obviously an important factor in the course of any operation. Animals die from incorrect dosage before the end of an operation and frequently before it begins. An experienced anaesthetist is,

1

therefore, essential. At the same time practical experience shows that to keep a full-time specialist anaesthetist for dogs is not always possible, and where there is such a specialist, there is always the question of who is to replace him when he is absent temporarily. Junior laboratory assistants do not usually have any special training for this work. The anaesthetist cannot be replaced by a qualified research worker, first, because this is not the work for which such workers have been appointed and, secondly, it is seldom possible to find such "selfless" individuals who, apart from one or two operations, will agree to undertake continued participation in such "dull" work as the administration of anaesthetics.

Not infrequently, therefore, the physiologist finds himself in a difficult position. The writer of these lines found himself in just such a position. In August 1956 I had to perform operations almost daily but there was no anaesthetist. The other workers in my laboratory were all away on leave. There were no scientific workers in neighbouring laboratories in a position to or willing to take a regular part in my operations. No help could be obtained anywhere until finally we constructed a very simple apparatus for ether anaesthesia, which freed us for all time from all these difficulties and defects and enabled us to dispense with one individual, the anaesthetist, who usually occupies the best position at the operating table, at the head of the dog, and hampers the surgeon during operation.

Description of the Apparatus for Ether Anaesthesia

The outward appearance of the apparatus is shown in Figure 1. The metal tube *16* with the screw *17* is fixed on the tripod *18*. The metal rod *1* slides in the tube and can be raised to various heights. The rod carries a wooden board *2*, 45 cm high and 12 cm wide. The support *4* is attached to the upper end of the board and on this is placed the glass jar *3* of capacity 400 ml and with a stopper through which passes the capillary glass tube *5*. The outlet tube *6* at the bottom of the jar is closed by a stopper through which passes a metal tube 3 mm in diameter and 4 cm long with the rubber tube *7* attached, the other end of the latter passing under the arm *A* of the lever *8* and through an oblique opening to the front of the board *2* (see Fig. 1, b). The weight *10* is so placed on the end of the arm

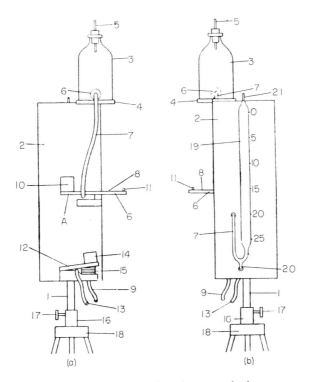

Fig. 1. Apparatus for ether anaesthesia.

a—view from behind. b—view from in front. *1*—metal rod. *2*—wooden board. *3*—glass jar. *4*—support. *5*—glass capillary tube. *6*—outlet tube of the jar. *7*—rubber tubing. *8*—simple lever. *9*—outlet tube from the "concertina" cylinder. *10*—weight (on simple lever). *11*—button. *12*—2nd type lever. *13*—rubber tubing going to the mask. *14*—weight (on 2nd type lever). *15*—"concertina" cylinder. *16*—metal tube. *17*—screw. *18*—tripod. *19*—burette. *20*—glass three-way connection. *21*—capillary glass tube. *A*, *B*—arms of the simple levers.

A that the rubber tube is completely compressed. Pressure on the button *11* on the other end of the lever (arm *B*) raises the weight and frees the rubber tube from pressure. On the rear of the board below the lever just described there is a 2nd type lever *12*, under which, nearer to the fulcrum, the rubber tube *13* emerges. The weight *14* is placed on the upper surface of the end of the lever and below is attached the cylinder *15* which, when inflated, raises the load and frees the rubber tube *13* connected with the ether mask.

The concertina cylinder *15* is connected by a long tube *9* with a rubber bulb which is placed under a foot piece (see Fig. 4, *4*).

The burette *19* with its scale (each division equals 1 ml) is seen on the front of the apparatus, its upper end ending in a capillary tube *21* and the lower end, 3 mm in diameter, being connected by a short rubber tube with the glass three-way connection *20*, another end of which is connected with the rubber tube *7* emerging through the board from its posterior side and the third with the rubber tube *13* going to the mask.

Figure 2 shows the metal mask *1*, which is shaped like a truncated cone divided in the medial plane, and is 9 cm in length (the dog lies on its abdomen). The radius of the anterior wall of the mask is 4 cm and that of the opening in the posterior wall 8 cm. On the undersurface there are the semicircular opening *4* for the upper incisors, a circular opening *6* for one canine tooth and a longer opening for the other upper canine. This opening makes it possible for both canines to emerge whatever the width of the dog's upper jaw.

Figure 3 shows a side view of the mask. A leather collar *2* (2 cm in width) is stitched to the edge of the posterior opening and to this is attached the draw-cord *3*. The metal tube *4*, 3 mm in diameter, is soldered to the upper surface of the mask, runs on to the anterior wall and, reaching its centre, passes back through an oblique opening in the anterior wall into the interior of the mask, where it bends upwards and slightly forwards so that the opening of the tube is not immediately under the dog's nose. In addition to the terminal opening this inner part of the tube has four other openings 1 mm in diameter, two on each side of the tube. Two are at a distance of 3 mm and the other two 6 mm from the end of the tube. There are

three openings of the same size in the upper wall of the mask
1 cm back from its anterior edge. The outer end of the metal
tube *4* is connected with the rubber tube *6* going to the burette
(Fig. 1, *19*). Cotton wool filling the space between the posterior
surface of the anterior wall and the dog's nose can be seen
within the mask.

Figure 4 is a longitudinal
section of the foot piece and
under it is the rubber bulb *1*
with rubber tube *5* going to the
cylinder, housed in a shallow
open box *2* on the base board
3. Figure 5 gives a general
view of the apparatus before
operation.

Fifteen minutes after the
injection of morphia, the dog
is anaesthetized with ether,
given with an ordinary mask.
After complete preparation in
the pre-operation room, the dog
is brought into the operation
theatre, placed on and bound to
the table. The upper jaw is
raised, the incisor and canine
teeth are covered with cotton
wool and the mask is applied.
The teeth covered with cotton
wool project through the openings *4*, *5* and *6* (Fig. 2), and the
openings are firmly plugged

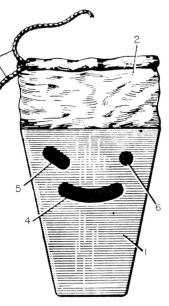

Fig. 2. Metal mask for anaesthesia
(seen from below).

1—metal mask. *2*—leather collar.
3—"tobacco-pouch" drawstring.
4—curved opening. *5*—elongated
opening. *6*—circular opening.

thereby. The mask is fixed on the upper jaw by means of the
cord passing through the leather collar on the upper edge of the
mask. When the cord is tightened, the collar grasps the upper
jaw firmly. The dog's mouth cavity is filled with cotton wool to
close the pharynx so that its respiration becomes completely
nasal and the air drawn through the mask into the trachea is
mixed with ether. From now on, the anaesthesia is looked after

by the theatre sister who can cope with it without difficulty while at the same time carrying out other duties connected with the operation.

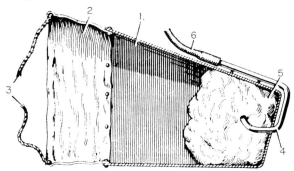

Fig. 3.   Longitudinal section of the mask for anaesthesia
(seen from the side).
1—metal mask. *2*—leather collar. *3*—drawstring. *4*—metal tube. *5*—wool.
6—rubber tubing from burette.

The sister places a sterile piece of gauze on the button (Fig. 1, *11*) and, pressing on the lever, fills the burette *19* with

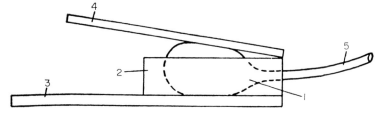

Fig. 4.   Longitudinal section of the pedal.
1—rubber bulb. *2*—wooden box. *3*—baseboard. *4*—pedal. *5*—rubber
tubing.

ether. Then, whenever required, she depresses the pedal with her foot, thereby removing the pressure from the rubber bulb and inflating the concertina cylinder *15* so that the required quantity of ether can reach the mask. On each occasion the sister presses button *11* to refill the burette.

It will be seen that this apparatus is very simply controlled.

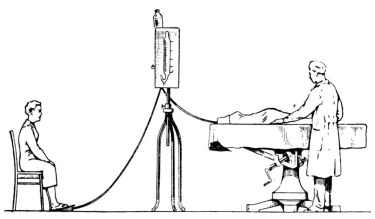

Fɪɢ. 5.　General view of the arrangement.

It should, however, be noted that, despite the simple construction of the apparatus and the enormous convenience it affords during operation, it did not occur to us to construct it until acute need for it arose as a result of a concatenation of circumstances, so that one cannot but recall the wisdom of the proverb—necessity is the mother of invention.

When an operation has to be carried out in the nasal region, the ether anaesthetic is administered to the dog through the mouth by means of another apparatus (Fig. 6), somewhat different from that described. A metal tube *2*, 3 mm in diameter, passes into another metal tube *1*, 4 cm long and 8 mm in diameter, and emerges at right angles through an opening in the middle of the latter tube, the projecting part being 7 cm long. 1 cm from the end of this

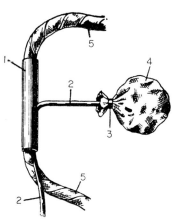

Fɪɢ. 6.　Apparatus for ether anaesthesia administered through the mouth. *1*—wide metal tube. *2*—narrow metal tube. *3*—ring on tube. *4*—gauze-covered ball of cotton-wool. *5*—gauze cord.

B

tube *2* there is a ring to which is attached a ball of cottonwool
covered with two layers of gauze *4*. Tube *2* is soldered to tube *1*
at its point of exit. A twisted band of gauze *5* passes through tube
1. During an operation the free end of tube *2* is connected by
rubber tubing to the burette of the apparatus described earlier
(Fig. 1, *19*).

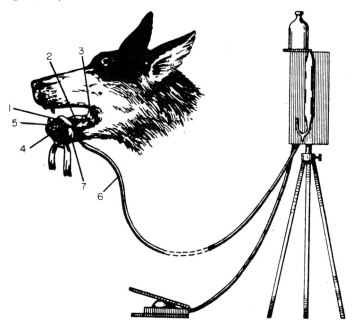

FIG. 7.   General view before operation with anaesthesia administered
through the mouth.
1—wide metal tube. *2*—narrow metal tube. *3*—cotton-wool covering up the
gauze-wool ball and closing the dog's pharynx. *4*—lower canine tooth.
5—tongue. *6*—rubber tubing from burette. *7*—gauze cord.

Figure 7 shows that tube *1* is placed behind the canine
teeth of the lower jaw and is fixed in this position by the gauze
band, which is tied below the lower jaw. The end of tube *2*
with the gauze-covered wool ball *3* is placed on the upper
surface of the tongue *5* opposite the larynx. The mouth cavity
in front of the ball is packed lightly with wool and the dog's

nostrils are closed with pledgets of wool to limit nasal respiration.

Construction of the Apparatus for Opening the Dog's Mouth

The wooden board *1* is 70 cm long, 30 cm wide and 2 cm thick (Figs. 8 and 9). Two metal rods 8 mm in diameter and 50 cm high *2* are fixed rigidly in the board 8 cm from the

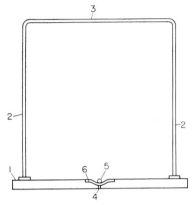

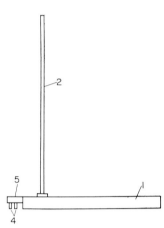

FIG. 8. Apparatus for opening the dog's mouth in operations for exteriorization of tongue segments (seen from front).
1—wooden board. *2*—metal rods. *3*—connecting rod. *4*—metal pins. *5*—metal rod in the anterior edge of the board. *6*—metal plate.

FIG. 9. Side view of the apparatus shown in Fig. 8 (same notation).

anterior edge and 2 cm from the sides, and the upper ends of these rods are firmly connected by the metal rod *3*, 8 mm in diameter. The metal rod *5*, 8 mm in diameter, projects for a distance of 4 cm from the middle of the anterior edge of the board. A metal plate 5 cm long, 4 cm wide and 2 mm thick, is bent at right angles to its length in such a way that the distance between the wings is 3 cm (Fig. 8, *6*), after which the projecting end of the rod is placed in the hollow of the plate and soldered to it. Two metal pins, 4 mm in diameter and 1 cm long, are soldered on to the convexity of the plate; the distance of the first pin from the front edge of the plate is 0·5 cm and the distance between the pins 1 cm (Figs. 8 and 9, *4*). The posterior edge of the board has a semicircular part cut out, 25 cm in diameter, and before operation the dog's shoulders are brought under this notch with the medial plane of the thorax vertical. At the front of the board the tip of the dog's lower jaw is placed

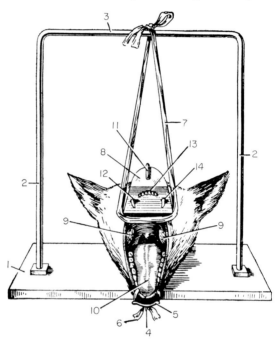

Fɪɢ. 10.   General view of the dog's head before commencement of the operation for exteriorization of tongue segments.

1—wooden board. *2*—metal rods. *3*—connecting rod. *4*—pins. *5*—metal plate. *6*—bandage fixing lower jaw to the plate. *7*—bandage opening the mouth cavity. *8*—anterior wall of the mask. *9*—tonsils. *10*—tongue. *11*—metal tube of mask. *12*—round opening in mask. *13*—curved opening. *14*—elongated opening.

in the groove formed by the bent plate and a sterile bandage *6* is drawn tight behind the canine teeth of the lower jaw and tied (Fig. 10) between the pins. This fixes the lower jaw rigidly. A second bandage *7* passes transversely under the upper jaw in front of the secondary teeth and behind the lower posterior edge of the mask. The two ends of the bandage are brought over the cross piece from opposite sides, are drawn as tight as possible and tied over the cross piece. The mouth is then cleared of saliva with pledgets of wool, washed with water (the water is expressed from pieces of wool or is allowed to flow from an irrigator through a rubber tube with a nozzle) and is then wiped dry, after which the tongue and the entire mouth cavity as far as the larynx are wiped with alcohol. A sterile sheet is placed over the dog and a sterile towel or sheet is placed under the lower jaw. Pieces of sterile wool are inserted into the pharynx until it is filled in order to restrict oral respiration and intensify the inhalation of anaesthesia. A start is then made with the operation, which can be carried out in two ways.

Operation for Exteriorization of the Mucous Membrane of Symmetrical Segments of the Tongue

The dog is given a subcutaneous injection of morphine hydrochloride 1 mg/2 kg in 1 per cent solution 15 min before anaesthesia. Ether is used for anaesthesia (for the technique see above). The lower jaw is shaved over an area limited anteriorally and laterally by the edges of the lower lips and behind by a transverse line at the level of the cricoid cartilage, which projects under the skin and can be readily palpated. The dog is then transferred to the operation table and placed on its abdomen with the paws tied to the edges of the table; the mouth is then opened.

First Method of Preparing Symmetrical Segments of the Posterior Part of the Tongue for Exteriorization

The lines of incision on the upper surface of the tongue are marked out by sutures (black for better visibility). A thread, inserted into an intestinal needle, is passed through the mucous membrane of the tongue. The first insertion of the needle is made on the left border of the tongue at a point on a transverse line 8 mm anterior to the most anterior circumvallate papilla. In the dog there are usually two pairs of circumvallate papillae, one on each side of the middle line. Two of the papillae lie close to the middle line and the other two somewhat more laterally. The two pairs are not symmetrically placed: the right pair is slightly anterior in some dogs and the left pair in others. The anterior transverse line of incision is determined by the position of the most anterior papilla. The second stitch is made at the junction between the lower and middle third of the palatoglossal arch of the corresponding side and the third, in the perpendicular dropped from the middle of the tonsil to the upper surface of the tongue, at a point the same height above the upper surface of the tongue as the second stitch. Another stitch is made at right angles to the midline to reach a point 2 mm away from the midline and the suture is then carried forward over the upper surface of the tongue parallel to the midline to the transverse line already mentioned. In inserting the stitches in the tongue the length of suture is short (2–3 mm) under the mucosa and longer over the mucosa (20–30 mm). The suture is then turned laterally and it ends at the place of the first insertion of the needle, so that the two ends of the thread (length 5 cm) are now free at this point. The lines of incision on the other half of the upper surface of the tongue are marked out with thread in the same order (Fig. 11). An incision is then made in the mucous membrane of the floor of the mouth. The incision starts on the edge of the tongue (at right angles to it) from a point 2 mm anterior to a line passing through

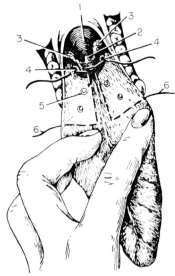

FIG. 11. Marking out of the incision lines in the first method for preparation of symmetrical segments of the posterior part of the tongue.

1—soft palate. *2*—epiglottis. *3*—palatine tonsil. *4*—joint between inferior and middle cornua. *5*—circumvallate papillae. *6*—threads marking the lines of incision.

the anterior thread and runs towards the inner surface of the body of the mandible. The incision divides successively the mucous membrane on the undersurface of the tongue and floor of the mouth cavity over the hypoglossal and lingual nerves and Wharton's duct, ending 6 mm from the point of attachment of the mucosa to the inner surface of the body of the mandible. The second incision in the mucosa starts from the same point and runs backward along the edge of the tongue to

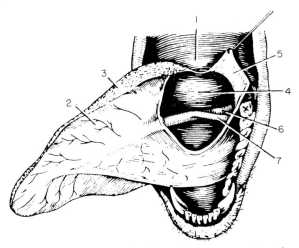

Fig. 12.   View of the tongue after incision of the mucosa on its under surface. *1*—soft palate. *2*—under surface of the tongue. *3*—margin of the upper surface of the tongue. *4*—styloglossus. *5*—edge of the divided mucosa drawn upwards. *6*—hypoglossal nerve. *7*—lingual nerve.

the point where the palatoglossal fold joins the edge of the tongue. The mucosa of the segment between the two incisions is then dissected off. As over a small area in the angle between the incisions the mucosa is firmly adherent to the underlying tissue, it has to be separated with scissors. Over its remaining extent the mucous membrane is easily separated with a blunt instrument, so that a cavity similar in shape to the coniform cavity between the tongue and the inner surface of the ramus of the mandible is rapidly formed, with its apex directed backwards. Above, this cavity is limited by the mucous mem-

brane and below by the muscles in the floor of the mouth
cavity, in which Wharton's duct, the hypoglossal and lingual
nerves and the styloglossus muscle are visible (Fig. 12). The
cavity is then enlarged backwards to a distance of 3 cm posterior
to the inferior cornu of the hyoid bone, the lingual nerve,
Wharton's duct and the sublingual salivary gland being moved

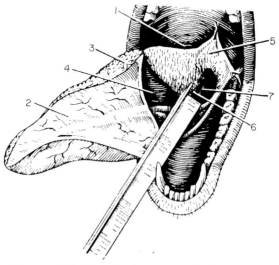

Fig. 13.   Tongue with the styloglossus muscle drawn downwards after
dissection of the glossopharyngeal nerve.
1—soft palate. *2*—under surface of the tongue. *3*—margin of the upper
surface of tongue *4*—styloglossus (drawn downwards). *5*—edge of the
divided mucosa drawn upwards. *6*—glossopharyngeal nerve. *7*—middle
cornu.

laterally from the styloglossus muscle. The anterior superior
edge of the mucosa is separated and drawn upwards and is
attached by a first stitch to the mucous membrane of the hard
palate at a point 1 cm medial and posterior to the last upper
molar tooth and a second suture 1 cm lateral and posterior
to this tooth. The lateral surface of the styloglossus muscle is
thus freed from the overlying tissues in the region of the middle
cornu of the hyoid bone (Fig. 12). With a curved dissecting
needle, this muscle is then separated along its upper edge from

the mucous membrane for a distance of 3 cm in the region of the middle cornu of the hyoid bone so that the latter becomes clearly visible. The styloglossus muscle is drawn downwards with a blunt hook (Fig. 13) to expose the middle cornu of the hyoid bone, and medial to this, in the submucous tissue of the mouth cavity, the glosso-pharyngeal nerve running anteriorly into the substance of the tongue. The nerve is separated from the surrounding tissue with a curved dissecting needle for a distance of 3 cm backwards from the point where it enters the substance of the tongue. This dissection of the nerve is the most difficult part of the operation: the nerve at this point is comparatively small and is quite firmly adherent to the submucous connective tissue, from which it differs little in colour. Not infrequently, in the course of the dissection the connective tissue becomes divided up longitudinally to form long delicate connective tissue strands which may easily be taken for the nerve. Landmarks become even more difficult to distinguish because of the capillary haemorrhage which frequently accompanies this operation. Consequently, some training in the dissection of this nerve in preparations is required if the necessary degree of skill is to be attained. Freed from the submucous tissue, the nerve is drawn downwards and the mucous membrane incision on the edge of the tongue is then continued backwards towards the root of the tongue to 2 mm

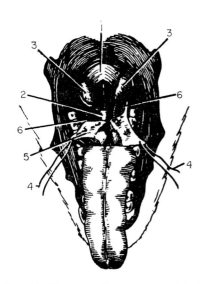

Fig. 14. Tongue with segments isolated. *1*—soft palate. *2*—epiglottis. *3*—palatine tonsil. *4*—tongue segments separated at the sides from the surrounding parts. *5*—circumvallate papillae. *6*—glosso-pharyngeal nerve.

behind the line of the inserted suture; the incision is then turned at a right angle to run parallel with the thread as far as the midline. The nerve on the right side is separated in the same way as that on the left and all the incisions in the mucosa of the tongue on the right side are symmetrical with those on the left. The incision running parallel and behind the suture at the root of the tongue on the right side joins the similar incision on the left side in the midline. The incision is then made deeper over

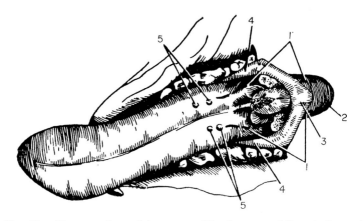

Fig. 15.   Upper surface of the tongue. The interrupted lines indicate the courses of the glossopharyngeal nerves.
1—line of glossopharyngeal nerve. *2*—pharynx. *3*—soft palate. *4*—palato-glossal arch. *5*—circumvallate papillae.

the entire width of the root of the tongue and the longitudinal muscles of the tongue (m. longitudinales superiores) and the longitudinal fibres of the mylohyoid muscle are divided.

The second transverse incision in the mucous membrane of the entire upper surface of the tongue is made 2 mm anterior to the anterior line along which the black thread was inserted, and 8 mm from the anterior circumvallate papilla. This incision is likewise deepened into the thickness of the tongue, so that the upper third of each styloglossus muscle is divided. The last incision in the mucosa of the upper surface of this segment of the tongue is made in the midline, between the transverse incisions just made, and is deepened to the level of the geniohyoid muscle (Fig. 14). The upper surface of the mucous membrane of each half of the posterior part of the tongue contains a pair of the main taste papillae (circumvallate papillae). Figure 14 shows the glossopharyngeal nerve running to the lateral angle of the tongue segment dissected out (6).

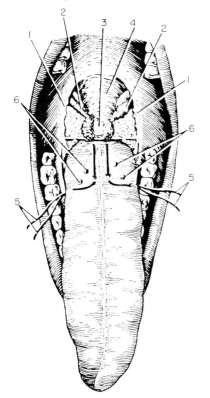

Second Method of Preparing Symmetrical Segments of the Posterior Part of the Tongue for Exteriorization

In this operation the glossopharyngeal nerve is not exposed and consequently the operation proceeds, as it were, blindly. But exteriorization of tongue segments by the second method is much easier and more rapid than by the first and the taste nerve is not damaged. In performing this operation the surgeon must above all remember the course of the sensory branch of the

FIG. 16. Incision lines for the second method of preparing symmetrical segments of the posterior part of the tongue.
1—palatoglossal arch. *2*—palatine tonsil. *3*—epiglottis. *4*—soft palate. *5*—free ends of the threads. *6*—circumvallate papillae.

glossopharyngeal nerve. It leaves the cavity of the skull through the jugular foramen, which lies immediately behind and medial to the bulla ossea. The nerve runs downwards, first in the submucous tissue of the nasopharynx at the junction between its middle and posterior third, and then in the submucous cavity of the mouth medial to the middle cornu of the hyoid bone, after which it disappears into the substance of the posterior part of the tongue. The course of the sensory branch of the glossopharyngeal nerve supplying the mucous membrane of the posterior part of the tongue in the region of the circumvallate papillae is indicated by the interrupted line in Fig. 15.

The dog's tongue is drawn forward and the lines of incision are marked out on the upper surface of the tongue with black sutures just as in the first type of operation. The stitches are made with an intestinal needle in the mucous membrane and submucous tissue. The length of each stitch is 1 cm. The needle is first inserted on the left border of the tongue in the transverse line across the upper surface of the tongue 8 mm anterior to the anterior circumvallate papillae. The second stitch is inserted at the junction between the lower and middle third of the anterior edge of the palatoglossal arch on the same side. The third stitch is in the mucous membrane of the mouth cavity at a point in a perpendicular from the middle of the tonsil on the same side to the upper surface of the tongue and at the same height above the upper surface as the second stitch. The fourth stitch is made at a point 1·5 cm anterior to the base of the epiglottis and 2 mm away from the midline. The thread is then turned forward and runs parallel to the midline as far as the transverse line already mentioned, where the next stitch is made, the thread passing laterally, and the last stitch is inserted alongside the first on the left border of the tongue. The free ends of the threads (10 cm long) are then carried to the outside. A segment of the same shape is marked out with sutures on the mucous membrane of the upper surface of the tongue on the right side (Fig. 16).

The mucous membrane of the upper surface of the tongue is then excised with fine scissors along the lines marked out. The incision begins at a point 2 mm anterior to the first point of insertion of the needle (see above), runs backwards parallel to and 2 mm external to the suture, and is then continued along the anterior edge of the palatoglossal fold to end 1 cm above the point where the suture turns. A similar incision is made on the right side. The mucous membrane on the undersurface of the tongue is then cut with scissors from the commencement of the incision on the left border of the tongue and at right angles to this border; this incision runs as far as the lingual nerve. The mucous membrane is then separated from the submucous tissue. The separation begins at the right angle and ends at a line joining the ends of the incisions. When the mucous membrane has been separated the segment of the submucosa exposed has the shape of a right-angled triangle. The separated

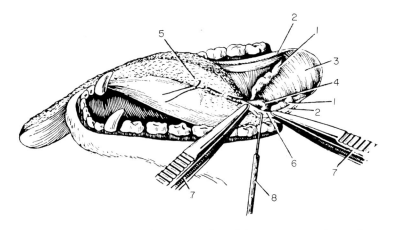

Fig. 17.   Commencement of the separation of the mucous membrane from the submucous tissue (second method of operation).
1—tonsil. *2*—palatoglossal arch. *3*—soft palate. *4*—epiglottis. *5*—lateral border of tongue. *6*—edge of the divided mucosa. *7*—forceps. *8*—curved dissecting needle.

mucosa is drawn back but is not divided. The lingual nerve is drawn laterally from the styloglossus muscle; the loose connective tissue between them is divided by a blunt instrument and the cleft so formed is deepened to the muscles in the floor of the mouth cavity. Attention is then turned to the point where the thread makes a turn from the anterior edge of the anterior palatoglossal fold, a point at the junction between the middle and lower third of the anterior border of this fold. With forceps held in the left hand the operator grasps the edge of the mucous

membrane at this point. The assistant takes hold of the mucous
membrane with forceps at the end of the incision, that is 1 cm
above the point where the stitch marking the line of the future
incision makes the turn (Fig. 17). With a curved dissecting
needle in his right hand the operator begins to separate the
edge of the mucous membrane from the submucosa between
the forceps; working from the edge of the mucosa, he penetrates
to a distance of 1 cm so that the submucosa is separated over
an area of 1 cm².

The operator's main task is to separate the mucosa from the
submucous tissue without damaging the latter to ensure the
integrity of the taste nerve lying superficially in the submucous
layer. The separated mucous membrane is incised midway
between the forceps parallel with the thread marking out the
incision. The forceps are moved forward, each grasping the
edge of the divided mucous membrane at the posterior end of
the incision, the edges are raised upwards, the mucous membrane
is again separated in the direction marked out by the thread,
an incision is again made in the middle and so on. Thus, the
separation is continued until the midline is reached. Finally,
a strip of submucosa 1 cm wide is exposed from the anterior
edge of the palatoglossal arch to the midline. This strip is
situated immediately behind the line marked out by the thread.
The mucosa on the right side is separated in the same way.

The two strips of dissected submucosa meet in the midline
and form a kind of horseshoe with the convexity towards the
base of the epiglottis. The edges of the incision in the mucous
membrane usually retract rapidly and become separated.
Consequently, the width of the strip after incision of the
mucosa is actually more than 1 cm. If the mucosa is dissected
from the submucous tissue as a thin layer, the taste nerve
(glossopharyngeal) which lies in the submucous tissue remains
undamaged. The operator then proceeds to separate the tongue
from the most posterior part of its root. The tip of the tongue
is covered with gauze and drawn forwards; with forceps in his
left hand the operator takes hold of the edge of the incision in
the mucous membrane on the upper surface of the root of the
tongue in the midline (tension is applied to this edge in the

line of the thread) and a perpendicular incision (about 1 cm in depth) is made in the muscles of the tongue. In this way the tongue is separated from the posterior part of its root and from the body of the hyoid bone. A transverse incision parallel to and 2 mm anterior to the anterior part of the marking thread is made in the mucosa on the upper surface of the tongue, dividing the upper third of the styloglossus muscles. The next incision in the mucosa is made in the midline between the threads and is carried down to the muscles in the floor of the mouth cavity. The tongue segments then assume the form shown in Figure 14 (the positions of the incisions in the mucosa are not identical at all points in the first and second methods).

The further stages of the operation are the same for both methods. The tongue segments are brought together, the tongue is covered with three layers of gauze, the wool plugs are withdrawn from the gullet, the mouth is closed, the dog is turned on its back and the neck is straightened out. The entire shaved surface of the lower jaw is painted with iodine, a sterile sheet with an opening, the edges of which are attached to the edges of the shaved area, is spread over. Incisions are then made in the skin and subcutaneous cellular tissue along the lower border of the body of the mandible on both sides. The commencement of each incision is in the straight line joining the body of the hyoid bone to the angle of the mandible. The incision begins at the middle of this line and runs posteriorly, parallel to the midline, for a distance of 4 cm. The wound is then enlarged by separating the skin and subcutaneous tissue. When the digastric and mylohyoid muscles are seen in the depth of the wound, the mylohyoid is divided through its entire thickness, this incision beginning 1 cm posterior to the commencement of the skin incision and 1 cm medial to the medial border of the digastric muscle and running backwards for 2 cm. When the divided edges of the muscle are separated the lingual nerve is seen running from the lateral side forward and approaching the hypoglossal nerve lying on its medial side.

It only remains to break through the thin layer of submucous connective tissue posterior to the point where the two nerves come close together in order to enter the mouth cavity. The tongue segment on the same side is brought out through the opening thus formed, is grasped with forceps by its lateral edge and is placed in the skin wound on the lower jaw; the lateral edge of the tongue segment is turned (in relation to the dog standing on its feet) laterally, downwards and then medially through an angle of 180°. In this way the lateral edge of the segment when in the mouth becomes the medial edge after

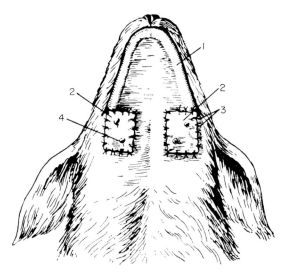

FIG. 18.   View of the tongue segments after exteriorization.
1—body of mandible. *2*—papillary surface of tongue segments. *3*—stitches fixing edges of papillary surfaces of the tongue segments in the prepared beds in the skin of the lower jaw. *4*—circumvallate papillae.

the operation for exteriorization, the medial becomes the lateral edge, and the mucosa (the papillary surface of the tongue, uppermost in the mouth cavity) is facing downwards in relation to the mouth cavity. The glossopharyngeal nerve enters the posteromedial angle of the exteriorized papillary surface of the tongue from the lateral side, crossing the middle cornu of the hyoid bone from the medial side and then running slightly laterally from this bone. A bed, corresponding in size to the surface of the exteriorized segment of tongue is then prepared in the skin wound, allowance being made for the fact that the edge of the mucous membrane must invariably be sutured over the skin margins, and the edges are sutured with knotted interrupted sutures. The sutures include skin, sub-cutaneous tissue and the edge of the divided muscle, and the needle then runs under the free edge of the mucous membrane on the exteriorized segment of tongue and is brought out through the mucosa, after which the ligature is tied. It must be remembered that if, at the posterior edge of the tongue segments and, to some extent also, on the medial border, the thickness of the tongue segment is included in the suture along with the free edge of the mucosa, the surgeon risks including the glosso-pharyngeal nerve in the ligature (thus interrupting the nerve) and depriving the tongue of innervation. Consequently, it is recommended that in this region the sutures should include only the free edge of the mucosa but elsewhere they may include the thickness of the muscle segment in the interest of safer suturing. The sutures should be about 4–5 mm apart. The same procedure is followed for exteriorization of the sym-metrical tongue segment on the opposite side (Fig. 18). The wound is then sutured, the ligatures are cut 2.5 mm from the knots and the edges of the wound are painted with iodine.

The dog is then returned to its original position and the mouth is opened wide for suturing of the wounds in the mouth cavity. At the points where the tongue segments have been exteriorized the glossopharyngeal nerve can be seen running downwards over the middle cornu of the hyoid bone and then running externally on its medial aspect. The sutures inserted for temporary fixation of the mucous membrane to the palate in the first type of operation are divided, and the edge of the mucous membrane is brought down. In the case of opera-tions of the second type, the glossopharyngeal nerves are not visible. Seven interrupted sutures are then inserted in the mucous membrane on each side of the mouth cavity, the line of suture being almost vertical and running forward from the palatine tonsil.

After division of the sutures (first method) the surface in-cisions in the tongue are sutured. The anterior edge of the

c

anterior transverse incision in the tongue (the posterior edge of this incision was exteriorized along with the tongue segments) is approximated to the edge of the incision in the mucosa bordering the epiglottis and sutures are inserted. This latter mucous margin is the upper edge of the posterior transverse incision (the anterior edge of this incision was exteriorized with the tongue segments). A surgical cutting needle with a stout silk ligature is inserted into the mucosa (at the base of the

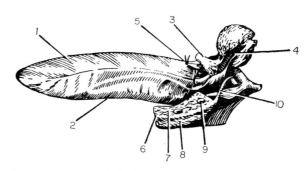

Fig. 19.   Tongue after isolation of the segments for exteriorization. *1*—upper surface of the tongue. *2*—under surface of the tongue. *3*—epiglottis. *4*—tonsil. *5*—stitches bring the anterior and posterior edges of the wound in the tongue together. *6*—tongue segment. *7*—papillary surface. *8*—under surface of tongue segment. *9*—circumvallate papillae. *10*—glossopharyngeal nerve.

epiglottis) in the midline through the submucous tissue and the remains of the muscles of the root of the tongue and then, directed upwards, passes under the base of the tongue incision to the anterior edge of the anterior incision, pierces the tongue muscles from below upwards and brings the ligature out on the upper surface of the tongue 4 mm anterior to the incision.

When the sutures are inserted in this way, the surgeon holds the needle pointing forward. He may, however, hold it pointing backwards, in which case the first insertion will be in the mucosa in the midline of the tongue 4 mm from the edge of the incision, or in other words this first ligature, like the others, passes through the same layers in the tongue but in the reverse direction. This method has a certain advantage in respect of free movement of the needle-holder in the mouth cavity. The ligature is not drawn tight as this would interfere with the introduction of the other ligatures, and Pean forceps are applied to its ends temporarily. A similar stout ligature is inserted midway between the central ligature and the lateral border of the tongue, together with four thinner ligatures, two midway between the stout ligatures and one on each side between the lateral stout ligature and the border of the tongue, the ends of each being taken in Pean forceps after insertion. Only then are the sutures drawn tight, the central ligature being tied off first.

The edges of the incision are approximated without any particular tension and the ligatures are cut off short; the sutured edges of the wound are painted with iodine. Figure 19 shows the position of the part of the tongue remaining in the mouth cavity with the left tongue segment prepared for exteriorization. The circumvallate papillae can be seen on the surface of the tongue segment and the glossopharyngeal nerve running to its lateral angle. The lower surface of the tongue segment conceals the pedicle of the latter. This pedicle, through which blood vessels pass to the tongue segment, is connected with the floor of the mouth cavity.

The dog is then placed in a room which has previously been disinfected with carbolic acid, and is placed on a lattice bed. If there has been considerable loss of blood, the dog is given subcutaneous saline, 20 g/kg heated to body temperature, on the operation table. The infusion is repeated on the following day. Saline is not injected if the blood loss has been small.

The dog is given nothing to drink or eat on the 1st day after the operation. On the morning of the 2nd day a small quantity of water at room temperature (3 ml/kg)is poured into the dog's mouth from a vessel. The dog swallows the water comparatively well. In the afternoon milk (5 ml/kg) is introduced in the same way and the same procedure is repeated on the 3rd day. On the 4th day the dog is given milk 3 times (morning, midday and afternoon), 20 ml/kg. On the 5th day it is given milk (10 ml/kg) in the morning and in the afternoon gruel-like food (minced meat, bread crumbs in soup or milk) is introduced into the mouth with a spoon. On the 6th day the dog begins to eat gruel-like food from a basin. It is not recommended that fluid food should be given, as tongue movements are not usually completely restored during this period and, in lapping, the fluid runs back into the basin from the mouth and the dog has to lap it again. This entails excessive movement of the jaws and may cause haemorrhage or displacement of the sutured tongue segments and the formation of an oral fistula. During this period milk or water is given as before from a vessel. The dog can be transferred to ordinary food two weeks after the operation.

Subcutaneous swelling in the region of the lower jaw develops on the 2nd postoperative day. There is continuous discharge of tenacious blood-stained saliva from the mouth. The mucous membrane of the exteriorized tongue segments is covered with a red crust. The swelling begins to diminish rapidly on the 3rd day and the scab on the line of sutures softens and separates gradually. The external sutures are removed on the 8th day as the edge of the mucosa is then firmly joined to the skin margin; the sutures in the mouth cavity separate themselves fairly rapidly.

Regular experiments with the dog can begin three weeks after the operation. As a test, the exteriorized surface of the tongue is stimulated with decinormal hydrochloric acid on the 6th or 7th day after the operation or in some cases even earlier. If the dog begins to lick its muzzle immediately when the mucous membrane of each of the exteriorized segments is painted, this indicates that the nerve supply to the mucosa of the tongue segments is intact. Occasionally, however, the post-operative period is protracted and active licking and excess salivation when the exteriorized tongue segments are painted with acid solution is only observed at quite a long interval after the operation. The reason for this would appear to be temporary damage to the taste nerve fibres during the operation.

Operation for Exteriorization of the Middle Parts of the Tongue

Symmetrical segments of mucosa from the middle section of the tongue can be exteriorized for the investigation of salivation from the glands on one side. The operation is much easier than the preceding but its after-effects for the dog are more severe. After the operation the middle part of the tongue remaining in the mouth is fixed to the floor of the mouth cavity. Only the tip of the tongue, over a length of 2–3 cm, can be moved freely and this is inadequate for the ordinary movements of the tongue during eating. The result is that the act of eating is very much protracted and, when the operation wounds have healed, some of the fluid food escapes from the mouth cavity and is scattered about. Even in this case, however, the dog can ultimately eat the food offered to it without assistance.

The dog is prepared just as for the preceding operation. The mouth is opened widely. An incision is made in the mucous membrane on the undersurface of the tongue from a point 4 cm behind the anterior border of the frenum and in the line separating the fixed part of the mucous membrane on the undersurface of the tongue from the remaining mobile mucosa on the floor of the mouth cavity. The incision runs for 2 cm at right angles to this line laterally and downwards. The posterior incision in the mucosa begins in this line at a point 4 cm posterior to the commencement of the first incision and runs parallel to it, also for a distance of 2 cm. An incision is then made in the line connecting the commencements of the two preceding incisions;[1] the edge of the incision is drawn slightly downwards.

Symmetrical incisions are made in the mucosa on the opposite side of the tongue. An anterior transverse incision is then made in the mucosa on the upper surface of the tongue and its muscles from above in the frontal plane passing through the anterior incisions in the mucosa mentioned. The transverse incision is of such a depth that it involves one-third of the styloglossus muscle; the posterior transverse incision in the tongue, made in the frontal plane passing through the posterior incisions in the mucous membrane, is of the same depth. After separation of the segment from the rest of the tongue a medial

[1]This incision thus follows the line separating the movable from the fixed part of the mucosa on the undersurface of the *tongue.*

incision is made down to the floor of the mouth cavity.

Gauze is placed over the wounds, the mouth is closed and the dog is turned on its back. A skin incision is made on the undersurface of the jaw from the middle of a line joining the body of the hyoid bone and the angle of the mandible forward for a distance of 3 cm. The wound is enlarged by separating the skin and subcutaneous tissue from the undersurface of the muscles of the mouth cavity to a distance of 1 cm from the lower border of the body of the mandible. An oblique incision 2 cm in length is made in the floor of the mouth parallel to the lower border of the body of the mandible. The tongue segment is grasped with forceps by its external edge and is carried downwards through the

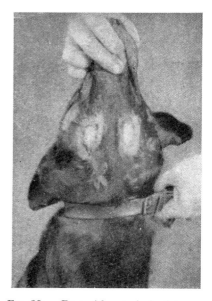

Fig. 20.   Dog with exteriorized tongue segments. The dog's head is raised.

incision to the outside under the lower jaw. After incision of the mucosa on the floor of the mouth cavity there is a passage from the external wound to the tongue segment. The lateral border of the segment becomes the medial border when exteriorized. The upper and lower edges of the mucosa on each segment of the tongue (these designations reflect the position of the tongue in the mouth cavity when the dog is standing) are sutured to the edges of the skin incision on the lower jaw. As the upper and lower surfaces of the tongue form an acute angle, the upper surface of the tongue will be directed downwards and laterally after these segments have been exteriorized and their edges sutured.

The postoperative care of the dog is as after exteriorization

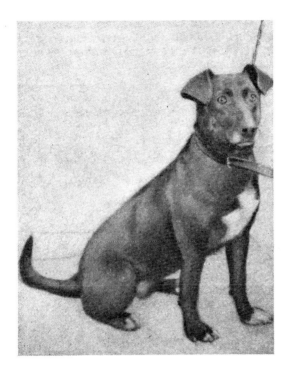

Fig. 21.   Dog with exteriorized tongue segments 9 years after the operation.

of posterior tongue segments. The wounds heal in much the same way. The mucous membrane of the exteriorized middle section of the tongue is liable to dry and its superficial layers are constantly being shed in the form of thin scales. To prevent this it is sufficient to paint the mucosa thinly with fish oil once every two days. It will then retain its normal pink colour and constant sensitiveness.

When the mucous membrane of exteriorized segments from the middle part of the dog's tongue is stimulated, the salivary secretion and licking and swallowing movements observed do not appear to differ in any way from the effects produced by stimulation of the mucosa on exteriorized segments of the posterior part of the tongue. We have, however, abandoned this operation because of certain disadvantages, already mentioned, connected with the feeding of the dog. The operation for exteriorization of the posterior tongue segments was found more suitable for chronic experiments on dogs. It had no adverse sequelae. No abnormalities of any sort were noted in connection with eating or drinking, barking or in the dogs' general condition. Consequently, it was this operation which we subsequently performed on our experimental dogs. Figure 20 shows a dog with symmetrical segments from the posterior third of the tongue exteriorized on the skin of the lower jaw. Nine years have passed since the operation. Experiments in which both the exteriorized tongue segments and the entire mouth cavity were stimulated have been carried out continuously on this dog yet Figure 21 shows that there is nothing unusual in the dog's appearance.

It should be noted that exteriorization of symmetrical segments of mucosa from the posterior third of the tongue has no effect on the value of salivation developing in dogs when given ordinary food (Travina, 1952a, 1952b, 1953a, 1953b, 1954a, 1954b, 1958). The values of conditioned and unconditioned salivation in response to the eating of a certain quantity of meat-biscuit powder were determined in chronic experiments on dogs. An operation for the exteriorization of symmetrical segments of the posterior third of the tongue was then performed and, when the dogs had recovered, it was established that the quantities of both conditioned and unconditioned salivation and the viscosity of the saliva were unchanged after the operation. Apparently the removal from the mouth cavity of such a small segment of tongue did not reveal itself when the very large remaining receptive surface of the anterior part of the digestive tract, including the pharynx, was stimulated by food.

Thus, conditioned reflexes can be formed in dogs after exteriorization of symmetrical tongue segments by stimulation of the mucosa on these segments (separately for each side).

Conditioned reflexes could be elaborated in this same dog by stimulation of the entire mouth cavity with ordinary food. Furthermore, both food substances (meat-biscuit powder, meat, sausage, soup, cheese) and repellent substances (salt solutions, acids) are used to stimulate the mucosa of the exteriorized segments. If the substance is in solid form it can be applied to the tongue segment by gentle pressure and rubbing on the surface, and if it is in solution, a pledget of wool held in forceps should be moistened with the solution and the mucous surface painted. The most convenient unconditioned stimuli for daily experiments on dogs with exteriorized tongue segments are decinormal hydrochloric acid and 5 to 30 per cent salt solutions. These solutions can be used to stimulate the segments in two ways: (a) from close at hand, in which case the experimenter sits near the dog and paints the mucosa of the tongue for a certain period of time with a pledget of wool moistened with the appropriate solution; (b) from a distance, in which case the experimenter sits outside the room in which the dog is and the unconditioned stimulation is effected by means of an apparatus operated by pneumatic transmission (Fig. 22).

Before an experiment the circular metal plate is attached by means of Mendeleyev cement to the exteriorized tongue segment in such a position that the lingual mucosa presents itself in the opening *13* in the plate and the circumvallate papillae are opposite the end of the lever.

When the rubber bulb *8* is compressed, the concertina cylinders *7* and *15* are simultaneously distended. The former discharges solution through the siphon tube *3* and the latter presses the end of the lever *11*, with the open end of the siphon tube attached to it, against the mucous membrane of the tongue; consequently, the lingual mucous surface is moistened by the drops of the discharging solution.

Plates can be attached to both exteriorized segments at the same time and the segments can be stimulated in any order and any variation. Experiments in which the mucous membranes of the exteriorized tongue segments were stimulated with decinormal acid or salt solution did not produce any changes in the lingual mucosa; nor were changes produced in the mucosa by the fact that it was outside, and no longer in the mouth cavity.

The dogs operated on in this way live under the same conditions as ordinary experimental dogs: they are kept in a common dog-house and eat the same food. They are brought on a lead over the quite considerable distance from the kennel to the experimental room at any time of year and in any

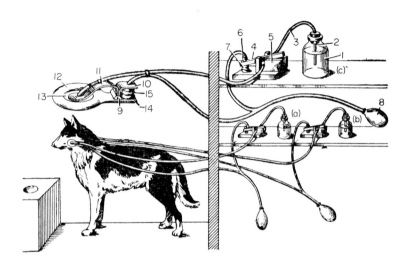

FIG. 22.   General view of the apparatus for stimulation of the mucous surface of exteriorized tongue segments.

a—vessel containing solution for stimulation of the left tongue segment. *b*—vessel containing solution for stimulation of the right tongue segment. *c*—the same vessel and accessory parts as in *a* and *b* shown in enlarged form. *1*—solution used for stimulation of the mucosa on exteriorized tongue segments (hydrochloric acid, common salt or broth solution). *2*—glass termination of the siphon tube. *3*—rubber part of the tube compressible by the lever. *4*—wooden lever. *5*—fulcrum of lever. *6*—weight attached to the end of the lever to compress the rubber tube. *7*—rubber concertina cylinder. *8*—rubber bulb. *9*—axis of the flat metal lever. *10*—short arm of the metal lever under which is a rubber concertina cylinder. *11*—long bent arm of the same lever through an opening in which the tubber end of the tube passes downwards and is attached to the undersurface by a thread. *12*—circular metal plate. *13*—circular opening in metal plate. *14*—projection on metal plate to which is attached the axis of the metal lever. *15*—rubber concertina cylinder.

weather. The mucous membrane of the exteriorized tongue segments is not affected adversely by these constant changes in atmospheric conditions. Colour, moistness and, what is most important, sensitivity remain unchanged.

We have made regular observations over a period of 12 years on one dog, called Mars, the first dog in which symmetrical segments of the posterior third of the tongue were exteriorized (from 26 December 1946). Over this period we have been unable to detect any changes in the external appearance of the mucosa of the exteriorized tongue segment or in the intensity of the salivary reactions when these segments are stimulated.

We give details of some illustrative experiments. The dog's left tongue segment was stimulated by painting three times with cotton wool moistened with 0.1 N HCl solution five times in the course of an experimental day at intervals of 5 min.

Salivation was recorded from the left salivary gland (Table 1).

TABLE 1. RESULTS OF PROLONGED OBSERVATION ON THE SALIVARY REACTION IN THE DOG MARS ON STIMULATION OF THE MUCOUS MEMBRANE OF AN EXTERIORIZED TONGUE SEGMENT.

Side of stimulation	Stimulus	Date of observation	Quantity of saliva (drops) on each stimulation				
Left tongue segment	0.1 N HCl	30 Jan. 1947	4	4	5	5	6
		30 Jan. 1956	6	6	6	6	6
		30 Jan. 1957	6	7	6	6	6
		30 Jan. 1958	6	7	6	6	6
		30 Jan. 1959	6	7	7	6	6

At the time of the last experiment (1959) this dog was about 15 years old. It had developed definite signs of senility (Fig. 23): its coat had become patchy, it was blind in one eye from cataract and it had become emaciated, but Table 1 shows that there was no change in its salivary function or in the sensitiveness of the mucosa on the exteriorized tongue segment.

The investigation of certain special problems in central

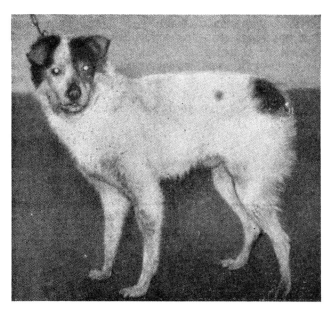

Fig. 23.   Dog in which tongue segments had been exteriorized 12 years
previously.

nervous system physiology requires the use of conditioned as
well as unconditioned stimulation of the receptive surface on
one side separately. Such unilateral stimulation is easily
achieved in the case of vision and cutaneous sensation. A special
apparatus has been constructed for unilateral acoustic stimulation (Fig. 24).

Figure 24 shows an ordinary sound-proof room for work
with conditioned reflexes. The chamber is made in a room with
main walls. Wooden boxes with side doors, lined with thick
layers of felt, are behind one of the walls (*1*). The box contains
a galvanized iron bell-shaped container with a removable
metal base on which are set the sources for various sounds
(metronome, bell, jar for gurgling sound, etc.). To the top
of the bell-shaped container is attached a double-walled rubber
tube (*3*). This is formed by inserting thinner rubber tubing
with an external diameter of 7 mm and an internal of 5 mm

into larger tubing 13 mm in diameter externally and 10 mm internally. The outer tubing ends 30 cm short of the end of the inner tubing. This is not shown in the diagram. From its connection with the metal bell-shaped container the double rubber tubing passes through an opening in the lid of the box, in which it fits tightly; it then runs through sloping openings in the walls SR and MW, in which openings it also fits tightly, and is carried to the stand for the dog.

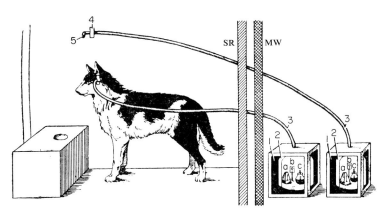

FIG. 24. General view of the apparatus for unilateral acoustic stimulation. *1*—layer of felt. *2*—metal bell-shaped container. *3*—double rubber tubing. *4*—metal plate. *5*—end-piece of rubber tubing. *SR*—wall of sound-proof room. *MW*—main wall of room. *a*—metronome. *b*—bell. *c*—source of gurgling sound.

The metal plate *4*, 4 cm² in area, is permanently fixed to the free end of the thin rubber tubing.

This plate is attached with Mendeleyev cement to the skin on the dog's head after the end of the thin rubber tubing, bent at a right angle, has been inserted deeply into the external auditory meatus (the bend in the rubber tubing is achieved by inserting it into a bent glass tube). The plate serves to prevent the tip of the tubber tubing *5* from moving in the meatus during an experiment and the tubing only carries the sound from the box with which it is connected.

A second box can be connected in the same way with the

other ear and alternating stimulations of the ears can be combined in a variety of ways.

A Modified Operation for Exteriorization of the Orifice of the Common Salivary Duct for the Submandibular and Sublingual Glands

The attachment of the cylinders for the collection of saliva from the orifices of the submandibular glands exteriorized in the dog by the old method presents difficulty. The orifices of the ducts of the submandibular glands are brought out together and are sutured to the skin on the anterior part of the lower jaw, which is narrow in this region. This does not allow of the simultaneous attachment of two cylinders.

We have, therefore, modified slightly the old method for the creation of fistulas of the dog's submandibular glands. Morphia is injected in the usual dosage (see above) and areas over the masseter muscle are shaved on both cheeks. The dog is anaesthetized, placed on the operation table and bound to it abdomen downwards, the mouth is opened wide (see apparatus for opening of the mouth). The mucous membrane under the tongue is incised in the midline between the openings of the submandibular ducts. The incision begins in the mental angle and extends for 5 cm to the anterior border of the frenum. The mucosa forming the edges of the incision is separated to a distance of 2 mm from the midline on each side; each edge is then taken up separately on two black ligatures, one at each end (the anterior ligature is 10 cm long and the posterior 5 cm).

Two incisions are then made in the sagittal plane on each side of the first incision. One begins at the upper end of the first incision and is carried laterally at a right angle for a distance of 1 cm, while the other begins at the anterior end of the first incision and is directed laterally and posteriorally along the medial surface of the body of the mandible and 5 mm from it (the length of this incision is also 1 cm). An incision is then made in the mucous membrane of the floor of the mouth connecting the ends of the two last incisions. This incision must be made with great care to avoid cutting the duct of the submandibular gland lying immediately under the mucous membrane.

A segment of mucous membrane in the form of a trapezium with one right angle is thus demarcated by the four incisions. The orifice of each Wharton's duct is situated in the midline on the side of the trapezium which runs parallel to this line. The opposite side of the trapezium crosses above the sub-mandibular duct. The two angles of the trapezium opposite to the angles marked by black ligatures are taken up on white ligatures 5 cm long. The ligatures of different colour and length enable the surgeon to identify the angles when the segment of mucosa with the orifice of the submandibular duct is finally being placed in the bed prepared in the skin of the cheek.

The next incision in the mucosa begins on the side of the trapezium crossing the duct and runs backwards along the duct to the point at which the lingual nerve crosses the sub-mandibular duct. The edges of the mucosa along the duct are separated back for 4 mm on each side to expose the duct. The duct with the segment of mucosa around its orifice is then dissected free from the surrounding tissue over the same extent (Fig. 25).

The duct on the other side is dissected out in the same way.

The tie raising the upper jaw is then undone and the dog's mouth is closed to enable the integuments of the jaw, which were stretched and displaced when the mouth was open, to resume their normal shape and position. The shaved areas on the cheeks are painted with iodine and the skin in the area on each side where the orifice of the exteriorized submandibular duct is to be situated is removed with scissors. Incisions forming an oval with a long axis of 3 cm directed vertically downwards, commence at the level of the upper borders of the zygomatic arch at the junction of its posterior and middle third (the short axis of the oval opening is 1 cm long).

The dog's mouth is again opened in the manner indicated, the operator grasps its lower jaw, which is covered below with sterile gauze, with his left hand, and the assistant draws the tongue away to the left. The operator holds a trocar for the right side in his right hand (Fig. 26).

The assistant threads the black suture on which the anterior end of the edge of the midline incision in the mucosa was taken up through the eye of the trocar and the trocar is introduced into the mouth cavity, its point being directed to the medial

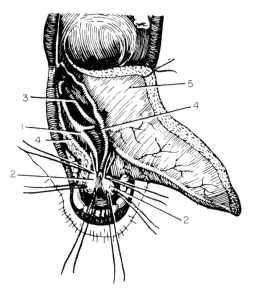

Fig. 25.   Position of the tongue during the isolation of the duct of the
submandibular gland.
1—Wharton's duct. *2*—segment of mucosa around its orifice (taken up on
sutures). *3*—lingual nerve. *4*—retracted edge of the incision in the mucosa
over Wharton's duct. *5*—undersurface of the tongue, drawn aside.

side of the last molar tooth posterior to the lingual nerve; the mylohyoid muscle is divided by the point of the trocar at its point of contact with the lower surface of the digastric muscle. The point of the trocar is then brought to the lower edge of the body of the mandible (without damaging the skin), is passed under the lower border of the mandible and the digastric muscle and is carried upwards to emerge through the skin opening on the cheek (Fig. 27).

The suture is withdrawn from the trocar and the latter is removed from the mouth. Traction is applied to the suture left in the skin wound to bring out the segment of mucosa with the orifice of the duct and the remaining sutures through the wound. The segment of mucous membrane with the duct

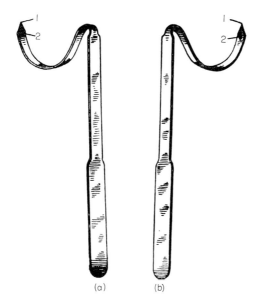

(a) (b)

Fig. 26. Trocars for exteriorization of the ducts of the submandibular glands.
a—for the right gland. *b*—for the left gland. *1*—point. *2*—eye.

orifice on the left side is brought out in the same way (with the trocar for the left side). The segments are covered with gauze and left for a time. Figure 28 shows the position of the trocar under the skin before it emerges (the skin has been removed from the dog's head).

The wound in the mucosa of the mouth cavity is then sutured with two continuous sutures. One is on the left side lrom the posterior end of the incision to the middle line (at the fevel of the angle of the mandible), and the second a similar suture on the right side, meeting the first in the midline. The

D

dog's mouth is then closed, the animal is turned on its back, its paws are fixed to the operation table and suturing of the mucosal segments with the duct openings into the skin of the cheek is started. The left segment of mucosa is set in correct position. The medial edge of the mucosa marked by the black sutures, now exteriorized, is turned backwards, its anterior extremity with the long suture being directed upwards and its

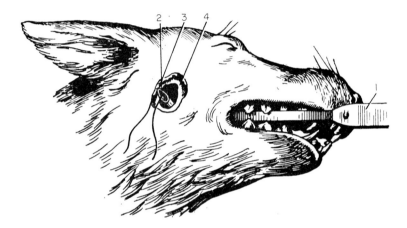

Fig. 27.   Position of the trocar with its point emerging through the skin
wound on the cheek.
1—trocar. *2*—eye of trocar. *3*—point of trocar. *4*—skin opening.

posterior extremity with the short black suture downwards. The skin opening is made to correspond in shape and size to the segment of mucosa and their edges are united by an interrupted suture. The knots are 5 mm apart. Figure 29 shows a segment of mucosa with the opening of the parotid duct exteriorized by the Glinskii method with the course of the duct after exteriorization shown diagrammatically (*1*, *3*); the diagram also shows the course of the submandibular duct after exteriorization (*2*, *4*). Figure 30 is a diagrammatic drawing of the parotid and submandibular glands (*1*, *3*) together with the courses of their ducts.

The duct of the submandibular gland on the opposite side

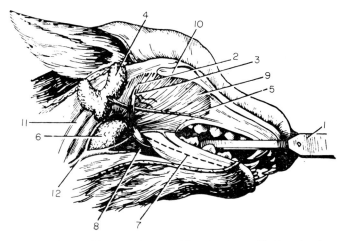

FIG. 28. Relative positions of the parotid and submandibular glands and the trocar under the skin.

1—trocar. *2*—point of trocar. *3*—eye of trocar. *4*—parotid gland. *5*—Stensen's duct. *6*—submandibular gland. *7*—Wharton's duct (projection). *8*—digastric muscle. *9*—masseter muscle. *10*—zygomatic arch. *11*—ala of the atlas. *12*—vein.

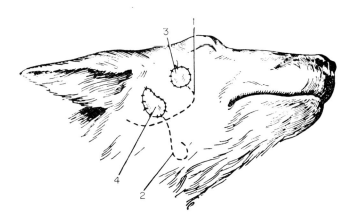

FIG. 29. Exteriorized orifices of the parotid and submandibular ducts *1*—Stensen's duct (projection). *2*—Wharton's duct (projection). *3*—segment of mucosa around the orifice of Stensen's duct. *4*—segment of mucosa around the orifice of Wharton's duct.

is then exteriorized. Care must be taken during the operation to ensure that the duct is not stretched. It passes under the lower border of the mandible and, if stretched too much, may be kinked by the edge of the bone so that the lumen of the duct is obliterated and the flow of saliva to the outside is arrested with the result that very soon (after two or three days) a cyst is formed in the submandibular gland. The same complication

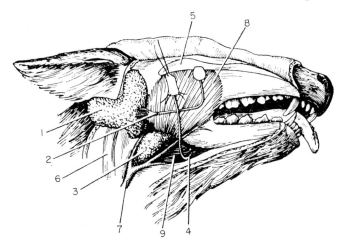

Fig. 30.   Diagram of the ducts of the parotid and submandibular glands in their courses under the skin after exteriorization of the orifices.
1—parotid gland. *2*—Stensen's duct (with segment of mucosa around the orifice). *3*—submandibular gland. *4*—Wharton's duct (with segment of mucosa around orifice). *5*—zygomatic arch. *6*—ala of the atlas. *7*—vein. *8*—masseter muscle. *9*—digastric muscle.

may arise if the mucosa around the orifice of the duct is not stretched out enough before suturing into the skin. The mucosa becomes folded and, when there is pressure from tissue swelling, the fold covers the opening of the duct, which later becomes completely obstructed and the outflow of saliva ceases. A cyst is also formed if there is twisting of the duct during its exteriorization. The rotation of the duct through 90° which occurs during the operation has no effect on the normal outflow of saliva.

The advantage of this method is that the two salivary ducts, the parotid duct and the combined submandibular and sublingual duct, can be exteriorized on each side at the same time. When exteriorized by this method, the orifices of the ducts are sufficiently far apart (see Fig. 30) for the simultaneous attachment of two cylinders. We have made continuous observations (for periods of more than 10 or 12 years) on many dogs operated on by this method and we have never noted any obvious abnormalities either in the weight of the dogs or in the state of the mucosa in the mouth. It follows, therefore, that the absence of the saliva from the main salivary glands (parotid, submandibular, sublingual) in the dog's mouth cavity has no obvious injurious effect on the animal.

Operation for Exteriorization of the Ducts of the Lachrymal Gland

All aseptic and antiseptic precautions are taken in these operations on dogs. Morphine hydrochloride 0·5 ml/kg of a 1 per cent solution is injected into the dog 15 min before it is anaesthetized (ether). The skin over the frontal bone, eyebrow and eyelid is shaved. The dog is then placed on the operation table, abdomen downwards, its paws being tied to the table; a wooden support is placed under the dog's lower jaw to raise its muzzle slightly.

The skin incision (dividing skin, subcutaneous tissue and muscle) starts at a point 5 mm above the junction between the middle and lateral third of the edge of the upper eyelid and runs in the sagittal plane for 2 cm. Skin and muscle are dissected up for 8 mm on each side of the incision to expose the orbital ligament and the attached connective tissue membrane. A longitudinal incision is then made through the entire thickness of the orbital ligament for 1 cm medially from the point of attachment of the ligament to the zygomatic process, both ends of the incision being continued forward at right angles as shown in Fig. 31.

The anterior part of the orbital ligament demarcated by these incisions is removed to reveal a part of the lachrymal gland, which can be readily recognized by its nodular structure and its more intense pink colour contrasting with the surrounding tissue. The connective tissue in front of the glands is then removed (this layer is generally thinner in front towards the edge of the upper eyelid).

The floor of the wound then consists of the submucous layer with, lying on its posterior part, the lachrymal gland above, and below, on the side towards the eyeball, the mucous membrane (conjunctiva of the upper eyelid). One pair of forceps is applied to the upper eyelid at the outer angle of the eye and another to the junction of the medial and middle thirds of the edge of the upper eyelid. The eyelid is drawn

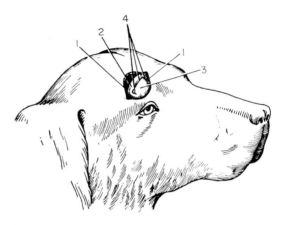

Fig. 31.   Incision of the integuments over the lachrymal gland.
1—separated edges of the skin and muscles. *2*—orbital ligament. *3*—tarsus.
4—incision in the orbital ligament and tarsus.

upwards and forwards so that the lachrymal gland becomes elongated as shown in Fig. 32.

Two sutures are then passed through submucous tissue and mucosa, their points of entry and exit being 1 cm apart and 7 mm from the edge of the upper eyelid; the midpoint between the entry and exit of the sutures should be opposite the middle of the anterior border of the lachrymal gland. The sutures are passed through the two areas separately. The needle is first thrust obliquely downwards (towards the eyeball) through the submucous layer and then through the conjunctiva. The point of the needle is then turned upwards entering the conjunctiva 2 mm away from its point of exit and in a line parallel with the edge of the eyelid, and then passes through the tissues from below upwards so that both ends are on the upper surface of the eyelid. A second suture is inserted in the same way at the opposite end of the line mentioned (see Fig. 32). An oblique incision (dividing the submucous layer and the conjunctiva) is made 2 mm anterior to the line of the sutures, after which the forceps are removed from the upper eyelid. The assistant

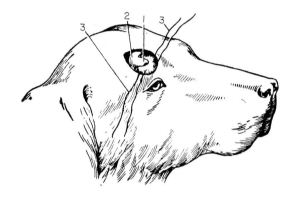

Fig. 32. Orbital ligament after removal of its anterior part. 1—lachrymal gland. 2—orbital ligament (remains of). 3—sutures picking up the submucous layer of the conjunctiva.

straightens the posterior edge of the incision by drawing the sutures laterally and anteriorally. The surgeon extends the anterior incision with scissors: he cuts round outside both sutures towards the superior fornix of the conjunctiva, each of these incisions making an angle of 55° with the anterior incision, so that they are directed to the superior fornix and slightly laterally and stop 0·5 cm from the fornix. The flap is then turned back (Fig. 33) and the final incision is made in the conjunctiva of the upper eyelid. Here, only the mucous membrane connecting the ends of the preceding oblique incisions directed to, but stopping 0·5 cm short of, the superior fornix, is divided.

This incision in the conjunctiva is thus 0·5 cm away from the superior fornix (Fig. 34).

Each edge of the incision in the conjunctiva is taken up on three sutures, one at each end and one in the middle. If the conjunctiva is relatively pale and little different in colour from the surrounding tissue, these sutures are inserted before the conjunctiva is incised, so that, even if the edges of the conjunctiva retract after incision, they are not lost in the submucous

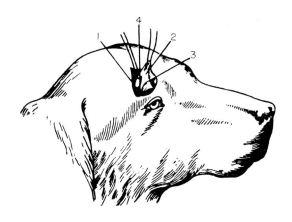

Fig. 33.   The isolated segment of conjunctiva turned upwards.
1—orbital ligament (remains of). *2*—segment of conjunctiva including the region in which the ducts of the lachrymal gland open (the segment is drawn backwards). *3*—superior fornix of the conjunctiva. *4*—eyeball.

layer and can be readily distinguished from it. Practically, it is better to use this second method in all cases. Each edge of the incision in the conjunctiva is then separated from the submucous tissue to a distance of 2 mm. The flap is drawn backwards by the sutures as far as possible, but without too much force, and the segment of conjunctiva is straightened out and placed in the bed of corresponding dimensions made in the skin wound. The segment of conjunctiva from the upper lid with the openings of the lachrymal gland ducts is thus facing upwards and the submucous layer with the lachrymal gland is lying on the remains of the orbital ligament. The upper eyelid

is everted and the edge of the incision in the conjunctiva near
to the superior fornix is drawn forward and sutured to the edge
of the incision close to the margin of the upper eyelid. The
knots are tied lateral to the eyeball and the suture ends are cut
short. A continuous layer of conjunctiva is thus formed over
the eyeball at the site of the conjunctival segment brought
out on the skin, and the upper eyelid is returned to its normal
position.

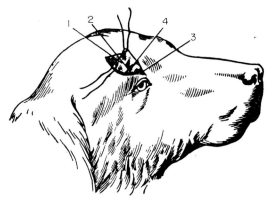

FIG. 34.   Exteriorization of the isolated segment of conjunctiva in the skin
wound.
1—the same segment as in Fig. 33, but now placed on the orbital ligament.
2—superior fornix of the conjunctiva. *3*—eyeball. *4*—incision in the
conjunctiva.

Then fixation of the flap is started. The edge of the flap of
submucous tissue and conjunctiva is made to overlap the skin
edge by 2 mm and is sutured in this position. The sutures
are 4 mm apart. The operation is completed by suturing the
edges of the flap incision in the skin on the upper eyelid with
three or four skin sutures (Fig. 35). The last stitch should be
1 cm away from the nearest edge of the exteriorized conjunctiva.

The orifices of the lachrymal ducts are not visible with the
naked eye on the surface of the conjunctiva and are difficult
to distinguish even with a glass. But when the conjunctiva of
the upper eyelid is incised in the manner indicated the orifices
of the lachrymal ducts are invariably found within these

incisions and when the flap is turned outwards and placed in the skin wound, the orifices of the lachrymal ducts will open on the surface of the skin.

Special treatment of the upper eyelid in the cadaver of the dog readily reveals the position of the orifices on the conjunctiva. The upper eyelid is removed along with the conjunctiva; the skin, orbital ligament and connective tissue are removed to expose the entire lachrymal glands. Numerous deep incisions are made with a pointed scalpel into the lachrymal glands. The

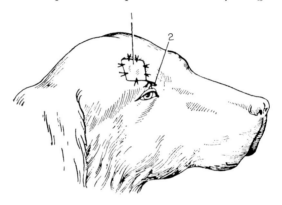

Fig. 35.   The isolated segment of conjunctiva carrying the openings of the lachrymal ducts sutured to the skin.

1—conjunctival segment with the openings of the lachrymal gland ducts is sutured on to skin incision. *2*—sutures in the remaining part of the original skin incision.

tap-controlled outlet at the lower end of a test tube is connected by rubber tubing to a vessel filled with fuchsin solution and a lachrymal gland preparation is placed over the mouth of the test tube with the conjunctiva facing upwards and the submucosa and lachrymal glands below, immersed in the fuchsin solution in the test tube. The edges of the conjunctiva are brought down over the edge of the test tube and a silk ligature is applied firmly below its mouth. The mouth of the test tube is thus firmly capped. The test tube is fixed in a stand. The tap of the test tube is then opened and the vessel containing the fuchsin is raised, so that the pressure in the tube is increased and the conjunctival membrane is stretched and bulges upwards, and when a certain pressure is reached, 12 to 15 tiny drops of fluid, clearly visible with a glass, appear in a certain position on the conjunctiva; it can be assumed that each tiny drop corresponds to a separate opening of a duct. The openings are situated close to one another in a circle of conjunctiva 6 mm in diameter.

The observation with the glass should begin before the pressure in the test tube is raised. There should be no further increase in pressure after the drops begin to appear, so that they can be counted. If the pressure continues to rise, the drops (at first very small) begin to increase in size and very soon run together to form a large drop which may run to the edge of the test tube. The mechanism responsible for the appearance of the small drops is readily explained. The lachrymal gland is immersed in fuchsin solution in the test tube. The branches of the ducts were divided at many points and their lumina opened by the preliminary incisions. When the pressure in the test tube is raised the fluid is driven into the incisions and through the ducts to their external orifices on the conjunctiva over the test tube. The fuchsin-stained fluid will ooze out in tiny drops on the conjunctiva, so that the position and number of orifices on the conjunctiva can be demonstrated.

The wound heals two or three weeks after the exteriorization of the orifices of the lachrymal ducts, the cornea and conjunctiva retain their normal colour and no abnormalities can be observed in the eye. The conjunctiva continues to be pink in colour and moist throughout the entire life of the dog.

The method employed for observation on tear secretion from the fistula is similar to the method for the observation of salivation. But the lachrymal gland discharges a volume of secretion which is 100 times less than that of the secretion of the salivary gland.

Removal of the Cerebral Cortex in the Dog

Haemorrhage is the most adverse feature the surgeon has to deal with in operations on the dog brain. Not infrequently it assumes considerable proportions and is the cause of the death of dogs either during the operation or one or two days after. The blood flows under the base of the brain, into the ventricles and into all the clefts, forming clots. When it is a question of operating on the brains of dogs which have undergone previous preparation, haemorrhage and death of the animals constitute a particularly sad experience for the experimenter. The result of the operation determines the result of the work previously carried out. With the death of the animal all the preliminary work is lost. It should be stated that the known methods for the prevention of haemorrhage (wax, ligature of vessels, use of preparations accelerating clotting of the blood etc.) do not always or all yield good results and their employment does not guarantee that the operation will have a favourable outcome. In searching for new methods to ensure the safety of dogs during operations on the brain, we gave first consideration to an important principle in surgery—the sparing as far as possible of bloodvessels, whatever their size, and the avoidance of areas notable for haemorrhage.

The preparation of the dog for operation follows the usual lines. The anterior limit of the shaved area of skin on the animal's head is a line through the anterior angles of the palpebral fissures, the lateral limit is at the level of the lower edge of the zygomatic bone and the posterior (on the upper surface of the neck) is a transverse line at the level of the anterior end of the spinous process of the epistropheus.

The dog is placed on the operation table, the shaved area is painted with iodine and the animal is covered with a sterile sheet with an opening, the edges of which are attached to the edges of the shaved area. The anaesthesia is continued with the mask described earlier. A skin incision is made along a line running posteriorly from the anterior angle of the palpebral fissure, parallel to the crista gallea, and an incision of skin and subcutaneous cellular tissue begins at the posterior border of the orbital ligament and runs to the superior nuchal line on the occipital bone. This incision is then deepened down to the bone through the thickness of the temporal muscle in a plane perpendicular to the surface of the skull. The edges of the incision in the muscle are turned upwards and downwards at the two ends, the reflections at the posterior end running along the superior nuchal line and the anterior reflections along the posterior border of the orbital ligament. Then the muscles in the edges of the first incision are separated off upwards and downwards with a separator and are drawn apart with retractors to expose the lateral surface of the skull as far as the crista gallea and below to the level of the commencement of the zygomatic process from the squama of the temporal bone; the operator then begins to open the skull, first with chisel and then bone forceps.

As the cutting of the bones of the skull along the midline and round the superior nuchal line is always accompanied by profuse haemorrhage, we make the upper and posterior edges of the opening in the skull 2 cm short of these lines to prevent this. It is impossible to separate the dura mater from the inner surface of the strips of bone remaining, as this too causes much haemorrhage, particularly in the region of the crista gallea. The frontal sinus on the same side is then opened. The upper part of the temporal muscle which has been divided and separated as far as the crista gallea, is then separated off from the entire length of the linea semicircularis to expose the lateral surface of the frontal sinus, which is opened, its superior, lateral and posterior walls being removed (Fig. 36), after which the dura mater is incised along the lower posterior and anterior edges of the opening in the skull and reflected towards the crista gallea, its upper border remaining undivided.

The bony septum between the sinuses and the attachment of the dura mater below to this septum are left untouched. This is to prevent the violent haemorrhage which develops when the dura mater is separated from this septum (see Fig. 36).

The skull is opened on the opposite side in exactly the same way if an operation is to be performed simultaneously on the other hemisphere. When the lateral parts of the skull and frontal sinus have been removed, the parts of the hemisphere visible are the anterior sylvian gyrus, the ectosylvian gyrus, the suprasylvian gyrus, the coronal gyrus, the lower part of the anterior and posterior central gyri and the orbital lobe (Fig.

37) (the names of the convolutions are as given by Ellenberger and Baum, 1891).

In addition to the convolutions a dense network of blood vessels, as shown in Figure 38, can be seen on the hemisphere. These vessels lie mainly on the external surface of the pia mater. In order to avoid severe and fatal haemorrhage we leave the pia mater *in situ*. We merely make three incisions between its vessels, namely in the middle of the anterior sylvian gyrus, over the posterior part of the ectosylvian gyrus and in the middle of the coronal gyrus, in that order. We work through

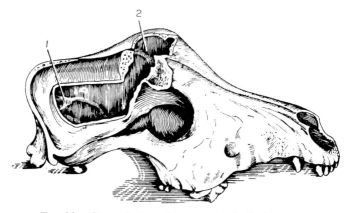

FIG. 36.   General view of the opened skull of the dog.
1—opening in the region of the temporal bone. *2*—opening in the region of the frontal sinus.

each of these incisions with a spoon and, with slow cautious movements, scoop out the gray substance to a depth of 1 cm. When the gray substance shown in the diagram has been removed, the pia mater falls away and the ectolateral, endodolateral and suprasplenial gyri descend slightly and come into sight. They are easily removed with the spoon under the pia mater through the incisions without damage to the neighbouring hemisphere, access to which is barred by the falx cerebri (its position is determined by feeling with the spoon).

The posterior part of the hemisphere (posterior suprasplenial and posterior splenial gyri) is then brought forward and

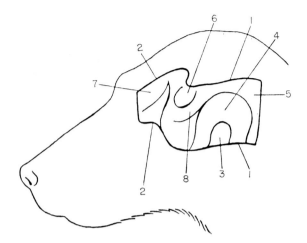

FIG. 37. Diagram of the cerebral convolutions exposed by the opening of the skull.
1—edge of the opening in the bone of the temporal region. *2*—edge of the opening in the bone of the frontal region. *3*—anterior sylvian gyrus. *4*—ectosylvian gyrus. *5*—suprasylvian gyrus. *6*—anterior and posterior central gyri. *7*—orbital lobe. *8*—coronal gyrus.

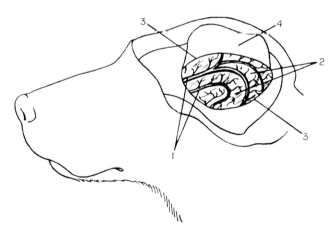

FIG. 38. Diagram of the vessels on the dog brain.
1—blood vessels. *2*—convolutions. *3*—edge of the opening in the skull. *4*—dura mater reflected upwards.

removed with the spoon from under the pia mater, under visual control. In this operation the hippocampus and the overlying optic thalamus, as well as the fornix and the caudate body are not exposed as they are covered by the remaining white substance, over which hangs the wrinkled pia mater with its well-filled blood vessels. The dura mater is brought down and covers most of the wound in the brain; this membrane is not sutured. Skin and muscle are then sutured with single sutures which can be removed easily when the wound heals. The single sutures prevent suppuration in the depth of the muscles, which often occurs when the muscles are sutured separately and are then under a second layer of sutures in the skin. One-stage suturing is effected more rapidly and shortens the time the wound takes to heal.

Removal of the Optic Thalamus

The dog is prepared in the same way as for the above operation and is placed on the operation table. An incision is made along a line from the medial angle of the palpebral fissure posteriorly parallel to the crista gallea. The skin and subcutaneous tissue are divided from the orbital ligament back to a transverse line through the posterior angles of the bases of the ears. The incision is deepened through the temporal muscle to the bone. This latter incision is made perpendicular to the lateral surface of the skull and runs from behind the orbital ligament to the posterior border of the skull (the incision of the muscles is not equal in length with the skin incision). Cross incisions down to the bone, 2 cm above and 2 cm below, are made at the ends of the incision in the muscle. The temporal muscle in the incision is separated from the bone to the crista gallea above and to the horizontal line passing above the base of the zygomatic bone below. This exposes the lateral surface of the skull, which is opened with a chisel, the opening then being enlarged with bone forceps. The upper edge of the opening is 1·5 cm away from the midline, the posterior is 1·5 cm anterior to the superior nuchal line, and the lower border is at the level of the upper border of the zygomatic bone. The anterior border lies 1 cm posterior to a perpendicular dropped from the end of the linea semicircularis. Thus, the frontal sinus is not opened.

The dura mater is divided along all the edges of the opening in the bone with the exception of the upper and the flap is thrown upwards. This exposes a large area of the convolutions (anterior sylvian, ectosylvian and suprasylvian gyri). An incision 1·5 cm in length is made with a fine scalpel along the posterior part of the suprasylvian gyrus and brain tissue is removed from this gyrus only with a spoon over the extent of the incision.

Two thin spatulas, placed in apposition, are introduced into the opening thus made in the brain and, their ends being separated to the width of this convolution, they are inserted deeper into the brain tissue in an anterior and slightly medial direction as far as the hippocampus which lies at a depth of 2 cm from the surface at the point of entry. One spatula is withdrawn and gentle pressure is exerted with the other on the lateral wall of the passage. The remaining part of the ectosylvian gyrus is thus displaced laterally to expose the entire posterior part of the hippocampus. The latter is divided lengthwise and the pulvinar of the optic thalamus, which is easily recognized by its bright pink colour, comes into view. An incision is made in the pulvinar and through this a small brain spoon is introduced into the optic thalamus and its entire mass is scooped out. After some practice the surgeon can readily feel the outer surface of the optic thalamus with the spoon, which limits the movements of the spoon like a capsule and ensures the safety of the surrounding brain structures, including the optic thalamus of the opposite side.

Transection of a Cerebral Peduncle and Removal of the Caudate Body

In this operation the optic thalamus is exposed as for its removal. The spatula is introduced under the pulvinar and pressure on the spatula downwards and forwards reveals the medial geniculate body; the cerebral peduncle of that side is then divided transversely with the spatula behind the medial geniculate body.

E

The preparation of the dogs for removal of the caudate body proceeds in the same way as for the preceding operations. An incision is made along a line running posteriorly from the internal angle of the eye parallel to the crista gallea. An incision through skin and subcutaneous tissue begins at the level of the orbital ligament and runs backward as far as a line joining the bases of the ears posteriorally. The temporal muscle is divided along the entire linea semicircularis on the side of the caudate body to be removed. The remaining part of the temporal muscle is then divided along a line parallel to the crista gallea and 1 cm distant from it; behind, the incision reaches the superior nuchal line. The temporal muscle is separated from the skull as far as the base of the zygomatic process.

The frontal sinus is opened and its superior, lateral and posterior walls are removed to expose the anterior part of the hemisphere; the lower part of the anterior central gyrus, the coronal gyrus and the orbital lobe are visible. The orbital lobe and the white substance to a depth of 4 cm under it are removed with a spoon and the head of the caudate body, thus exposed, is also removed. The spoon is then moved further back and slightly laterally to remove the remaining part of the caudate body.

Division of a Lateral Half of the Medulla

The skin incision begins at the level of the external occipital protuberance and runs in the midline to the level of the posterior end of the spinous process of the second cervical vertebra. The wound is deepened in the mid-occipital plane, first over the external surface of the squama, then over the membrane between the edge of the squama and the first cervical vertebra and over the spinous process of the second cervical vertebra between the splenius and the levator scapulae muscles. These muscles are divided by an incision from the external occipital protuberance along the medial half of the superior nuchal line and a separator is then used to expose the squama of the occipital bone.

The dog's head is flexed downwards, the membrane between

the squama and the first vertebra being thereby stretched, the second vertebra recedes and the first becomes prominent. The muscles are separated from the superior surface of the body of the first vertebra and from the spinous process of the second (the membrane is separated from the edge of the foramen magnum between the condyloid processes). The squama is then removed with chisel and bone-forceps along a line 1 cm posterior to the nuchal line, the condyloid processes being left intact. The posterior border of the cerebellum is exposed and is raised with a spatula. The tearing of the loose connective tissue at this point causes haemorrhage which is generally of short duration. The posterior part of the cerebellum is raised by cautious movement of the spatula upwards and forwards, uncovering the entire rhomboid fossa, which is examined with appropriate illumination from behind.

Raising the cerebellum with the spatula held in his left hand, the surgeon introduces a hook bent at a right angle (the length of the bend is 1 cm) under the cerebellum with his right hand. The point of the angled part is thrust perpendicularly into the floor of the rhomboid fossa in the midline at the midpoint of the diagonal down to bone. Movement of the point over the bone to the right or to the left divides the lateral half of the medulla on the corresponding side. The hook is removed from the brain wound and skin and muscles are sutured in the usual way.

The result of such an operation is unilateral paralysis of the skeletal musculature. The dog can no longer stand. When attempts are made to seize food, the dog's head sways markedly and the animal makes contortive movements in its attempt to turn over. The dog's head should therefore be held when it is eating. These dogs develop pressure sores rapidly and usually die from sepsis.

The danger area in operations on the medulla is the posterior angle of the rhomboid fossa, wounding of which causes arrest of respiration with cardiac activity remaining in a relatively good state. By employing artificial respiration we were able to keep one such dog alive for 8 hr but independent respiration was still not restored after that period.

CHAPTER TWO

EXPERIMENTAL SECTION

Latent Excitation

THE exteriorization of salivary and lachrymal gland ducts and of symmetrical segments of tongue makes it possible to observe the reflex reactions of each of these paired glands (salivary and lachrymal) in relation to separate stimulation of the corresponding receptive surfaces, the tongue segments and conjunctivae.

In addition to acid, solutions of common salt and, in special experiments, alcohol, broth and other food and repellent substances have been used to stimulate the tongue.

What is termed latent excitation remains for some time in the corresponding part of the central nervous system after stimulation of the mucous membrane of a tongue segment and, apparently, after stimulation of any receptive surface, even after the visible effect produced has ceased.

This phenomenon and term have long been known in physiology. The term is generally taken to mean a special state, the state of latent excitation, which arises as a result of subliminal stimulations. When first applied, a subliminal stimulus fails to produce any external effect but leaves behind a trace in the form of latent excitation, which is combined with subsequent similar traces produced by further applications of the subliminal stimulus so that a certain definite intensity of excitation is reached and finally, this manifests itself in the form of an external reaction.

Thus, the excitation arising before the development of the external effect has been termed latent. Subsequent experiments have shown that exactly the same state develops in the central nervous system after the end of an external effect. Consequently, on analogy with the former, the latter has also been termed latent excitation. There is no essential difference between the two. This problem has been discussed in detail in a work published by us under the title "The summation reflex" (Abuladze, 1949) and also in papers by Travina (1952a, 1955a, 1956a, 1956b, 1960).

These papers show that when, on the same dog and on the same day, a sterotype of acid stimuli is used in one half of the experiment and a stereotype of alimentary stimuli in the other half, then the same extraneous agent elicits an acid reaction in the "acid half" and an alimentary reaction in the "alimentary half". The only way in which this phenomenon can be explained is by the presence of latent excitation. It must be assumed that the application of the acid stimuli is followed by the development of latent acid excitation in the corresponding region of the central nervous system and that the extraneous excitation developing during this period in the central nervous system as a result of the action of the extraneous stimulus combines with the latent excitation to give an acid effect, or in other words, an acid summation reflex. Exactly the same mechanism produces an alimentary summation reflex when the same stimulus is applied after the alimentary reflexes, that is during a period in which there is latent alimentary excitation in the central nervous system.

Summation reflex experiments were carried out with exteriorized symmetrical segments of the posterior third of the tongue. In these experiments latent excitation was produced, sometimes on the left and sometimes on the right side of the central nervous system, by the action of an unconditioned stimulus on the tongue segment of the corresponding side (Abuladze, 1953; Gavrilova, 1954, 1960a, 1960b; Kolosova, 1959; Lapina, 1953a, 1953b, 1956b, 1957, 1958; Travina, 1953a, 1953b, 1954b, 1955a, 1956a, 1956b).

It was found in these experiments than when the extraneous stimulus was applied after stimulation, let us say, of the left tongue segment, the summation salivary reflex was on the left side and when the same stimulus was applied after stimulation of the right tongue segment, the summation salivary reflex was then observed on the right side.

These experiments demonstrated, first, that latent excitation was the basis of the mechanism in the summation reflex on one side and, secondly, that latent excitation persisted in the region of the central nervous system and remained on the side in which it developed.

The summation reflex in the presence of latent excitation is brought about by the same mechanism as the effect of a dominant focus. This is a fundamental point of similarity between the dominant focus and latent excitation. But these phenomena also differ in the details of their properties. The dominant focus is sustained by the effect of the stimulus when it is acting. Latent excitation on the other hand develops after the effect from the acting stimulus, and its intensity increases with increase in the strength or frequency of application of the stimulus.

The concept of latent excitation is not identical with the concept of tone as the latter is understood in physiology to mean the well defined state associated with muscular activity. Nor can it be identified with excitability as excitability can occur in nerve tissue both when there is no external effect and when there is activity of any kind.

As already stated, the outstanding feature of latent excitation is the absence of any visible external effect (gland secretion in our experiments) and the fact that it can only be demonstrated after the application of some external stimulus, the reaction being, it may be noted, non-specific, as it develops with any stimulus, conditioned, indifferent or unconditioned. For convenience in the discussion that follows, we can therefore distinguish two states of excitation, patent or declared excitation, which causes secretion, and latent excitation, in which case there is no secretion and the demonstration of its external effect requires special conditions. Latent excitation which has developed at a certain point may disappear rapidly but usually disappears gradually, the period of its existence ranging from minutes to hours (Gavrilova, Kolosova, Lapina, Travina).

We still do not know exactly under what conditions latent excitation can pass from the focus where it develops to another point, as for instance from one hemisphere to the other. Latent excitation does not itself appear to pass to the opposite hemisphere, and if an excitatory process is observed in this hemisphere, it can only be the result of a stimulus which is actually acting. The powerful excitation spreads from the focus of its development in one hemisphere to a focus on the other side and, when action of the stimulus ceases, latent excitation develops on both sides, on the side of the original development of the declared excitation and also on the opposite side, the side to which the declared excitation irradiated.

It must, therefore, be assumed that there is no direct transfer of latent excitation from one side to the other.

Our further experiments will show that latent excitation is an important factor in the production of many phenomena in the central nervous system.

Unconditioned Secretory Reaction of the Glands on One Side

Separate stimulation of the exteriorized tongue segment on each side and of the conjunctiva of each eye was used in the investigation of unconditioned secretory reflexes of paired glands (salivary and lachrymal).

When a weak unconditioned stimulus acted on one of any of the receptive surfaces, only the gland on the same side reacted.

For example, when the conjunctiva of one eye was stimulated the lachrymal gland on the same side reacted, and in the same way only the salivary gland on the same side reacted when a

TABLE 2. TEAR SECRETION ON STIMULATION OF ONE CONJUNCTIVA WITH WEAK HYDROCHLORIC ACID SOLUTIONS (0.5 N HCl). EXPERIMENT ON THE DOG EROS, 28 NOVEMBER 1957.

Left side		Right side	
Gland	Secretion (drops)	Secretion (drops)	Gland
Lachrymal	1	0	Lachrymal
Parotid	0	0	Parotid

TABLE 3. SALIVATION ON STIMULATION OF THE MUCOSA OF ONE EXTERIORIZED TONGUE SEGMENT WITH A WEAK HYDROCHLORIC ACID SOLUTION (0·5 N HCl). EXPERIMENT ON THE DOG EROS, 29 NOVEMBER 1957

Left side		Right side	
Gland	Secretion (drops)	Secretion (drops)	Gland
Lachrymal	0	0	Lachrymal
Parotid	3	0	Parotid

tongue segment on one side was stimulated. The strength of such stimulation was selected empirically by trying solutions of various strengths or by varying the length of time a solution of fixed strength acted. Tables 2 and 3 give the results of these experiments.

When the stimulation strength was increased a reaction appeared in the other gland also. Below we give experiments (on the same dog) in which a stronger hydrochloric acid solution was used (Table 4).

TABLE 4. TEAR SECRETION ON STIMULATION OF THE CONJUNCTIVA OF THE LEFT EYE WITH A STRONG HYDROCHLORIC ACID SOLUTION (0·3 N HCl). EXPERIMENT ON THE DOG EROS, 14 JANUARY 1958.

Left side		Right side	
Gland	Secretion (drops)	Secretion (drops)	Gland
Lachrymal	3	1	Lachrymal
Parotid	6	0	Parotid

These records show that, when the strength of stimulation was increased, the excitation irradiated from the point corresponding to the receptive surface stimulated to other points in the central nervous system, the irradiation being however selective: in the first experiment in which the left conjunctiva

TABLE 5. STIMULATION OF THE MUCOSA ON THE LEFT TONGUE
SEGMENT WITH A STRONG HYDROCHLORIC ACID SOLUTION (0·33 N HCl).
EXPERIMENT ON THE DOG EROS, 24 JANUARY 1958.

Left side		Right side	
Gland	Secretion (drops)	Secretion (drops)	Gland
Lachrymal	1	0	Lachrymal
Parotid	27	10	Parotid

was stimulated, the left lachrymal, left parotid and right lachrymal glands reacted but the right parotid gland did not react.

The same happened in the second experiment in which the stimulation started from a different point. The left tongue segment was stimulated and the excitation spread on the left side to the left lachrymal gland and on the right side to the parotid gland. The right lachrymal gland remained uninfluenced.

A clear example of selective irradiation was seen in experiments with a special form of excitation—sexual excitation (Table 6). It was found that whenever a male was brought into close contact with a female in oestrus, the male exhibited intense secretion from the submandibular gland but none from the parotid gland. No salivation was observed when the male was brought into the proximity of a female not in oestrus.

The experiment of 22 December 1957 shows that there was salivation from the submandibular glands only, while the parotid glands remained quiescent in the male dog when in the proximity of the female. It can be concluded that the sexual excitation which developed in a certain centre in the nervous system irradiated to other parts (salivary) selectively, involving only the nervous apparatus for the submandibular glands and not in any way affecting that for the parotid glands. It should be emphasized that in these experiments the male was 5–8 cm away from the female and that licking was not permitted. In

TABLE 6. SALIVATION (IN DROPS) FROM THE PAROTID AND SUB-
MANDIBULAR GLANDS IN THE MALE DOG (EROS) WHEN EATING AND
WHEN IN THE PROXIMITY OF A FEMALE.

Date of experiment	Action on dog	Salivation			
		From parotid gland		From submandibular gland	
		Left	Right	Left	Right
22 Dec. 1957	Brought into proximity of female during oestrus	0	0	13	20
31 Dec. 1957	Given meat-biscuit to eat	16	15	26	40
	Brought into proximity of female during oestrus after complete cessation of salivation	0	0	26	28
16 Jan. 1958	Brought into proximity of female not in oestrus	0	0	0	0

the course of an experimental day the animal was brought into this proximity a number of times (up to 30) at intervals of 2 or 3 min, but we were unable to note any reduction in secretion at the end of the experiment. It would appear that this secretory reaction is of the nature of an unconditioned reflex or a persistent natural conditioned reflex.

The experiment of 31 December 1957 was a control. The dog was first given meat-biscuit powder, the eating of which led to profuse secretion of saliva from all the glands simultaneously—parotid and submandibular. Ten minutes after the finish of eating, when salivary secretion from the glands had completely ceased, the male was brought up to the female so that its muzzle was 5 cm from the genital region of the female; there was a vigorous reaction of the submandibular glands only and the parotid glands remained quiescent.

A similar separate reaction of the submandibular glands also occurred when the male was allowed to lick or even to make connection with the female. The last experiment, that of 16 January 1958, showed that the salivary glands (parotid and submandibular) did not react when the male was brought into proximity with the female at times other than during oestrus. Examination of these experiments leads to the conclusion that one of the main conditions for the passage of excitation from the point of its development to another point is the degree of its intensity. Below we shall examine two further conditions for the transfer of excitation from one hemisphere to the other.

Experiments were carried out on dogs with exteriorized symmetrical tongue segments in which only parotid gland salivation was recorded. The excitation irradiated from one point in the central nervous system to the symmetrical point on the opposite side when there was latent excitation present in the latter, that is in the presence of the special state which remains in the central nervous system after stimulus action ends and after the visible external reaction in the form of salivation ceases. This latent excitation attracts excitation from the point on the opposite side to the focus of its development. Below we give details from the corresponding experiments.

TABLE 7. IRRADIATION OF EXCITATION (STIMULUS— 0·1 N HCl) WHEN THE RIGHT GLAND WAS IN A STATE OF REST. EXPERIMENT ON THE DOG DEVONKA, 2 NOVEMBER 1953.

Surface stimulated	Unconditioned reflex salivation from parotid glands in each 10-sec period (scale divisions)	
	Left	Right
Left tongue segment	140	50
	140	20
	70	10
	40	0

Table 7 shows that, while there was more salivation on the left side, there was also salivation on the right side, as represented by the values 50, 20, 10 and 0.

The right tongue segment was stimulated by painting with 0·1 N HCl for 2 sec five minutes after salivation on the left side had ended. This elicited salivation from the right gland in quantities of 60, 30, 10 and 0 scale divisions. When the left tongue segment was again stimulated for 10 sec (0·1 N HCl) 5 min after salivation on the right side had ceased, the right-sided salivation was then increased to 60, 50, 30 and 10 (Table 8) instead of 50, 20, 10 and 0 scale divisions (see Table 7).

TABLE 8.

Surface stimulated	Unconditioned reflex salivation from parotid glands in each 10-sec period (scale divisions)	
	Left	Right
Left tongue segment	0	60
	0	30
	0	10
	0	0
	150	60
	140	50
	60	30
	20	10

It is quite obvious that the latent excitation, which developed on the right side after the termination of salivation on that side, promoted the irradiation of excitation, i.e. transfer of the excitation from the left to the right side, on stimulation of the left tongue segment, so that a greater quantity of secretion than in the preceding experiment was observed on the right side.

The next condition for the irradiation of excitation from one side of the brain to the other is the presence of declared excitation in two points in the central nervous system, in our case symmetrical points. In these experiments excitation passed from the stronger to the weaker focus of excitation.

The experiments were carried out in several different forms. In one form we established the initial background of salivation for the left and right parotid glands separately in relation to the application of strong stimulation to one tongue segment and weak stimulation to the other. For example, one segment was stimulated with decinormal HCl for 10 sec and the other for 2 sec. The salivation had different values in accordance with the intensity of the unconditioned stimulus. On one of the succeeding days the stimulation of the tongue segments started simultaneously and the salivation was recorded from each of the salivary glands. This form of experiment revealed that salivation on the side of the weak stimulation was increased. The increase of salivation on the side of weak stimulation was assessed by comparison of the salivation with the value of salivation on the same side on the preceding days.

Another form of experiment was also used to demonstrate the transfer of excitation. The two tongue segments were not stimulated simultaneously. We first established the background salivation for the salivary glands of each side separately in response to stimulation of the corresponding segment of tongue. The right tongue segment was stimulated for 10 sec with decinormal acid solution. Salivation was recorded for each 10 sec period. The average value of salivation from the left salivary gland was 45–80–65–40–20–10–0 scale divisions. When the right tongue segment was stimulated for 2 sec, the average value of salivation from the right salivary gland, likewise read for each 10-sec period, was 40–30–15–5–0. On one of the next experimental days stimulation of the mucosa of the right tongue segment with acid for 2 sec was started 20 sec after the commencement of stimulation of the left tongue segment, at a time when the secretion was showing its maximum increase (80 scale divisions); in this case the excitation passed from left to right and there was increased salivation on the right side (75 scale divisions instead of the normal 40 during the first 10 sec). When 2 sec stimulation of the mucosa on the right tongue segment was added to stimulation on the left side 50 sec after the start of the latter (that is when secretion on the left side was beginning to disappear), the opposite happened: excitation passed from the right to the left side and the almost disappearing excitation on the left side was increased again (30 or 20 divisions instead of the usual 10).

Excitation passing from left to right and from right to left, depending on the strength relationships between the excitatory processes which developed at the particular moment on the two sides of the brain, could be observed in the same dog in the course of the same experimental day.

The word "transfer" or "passage" which we use frequently and which the reader will still meet with, must not be understood in its literal sense, namely that excitation passes from one side to the other in the way that fluid moves between communicating vessels at different heights. When the reaction on the side of weak excitation increases, this does not always cause the reaction on the side of strong excitation to be reduced to the same extent. At the same time, direct transfer, as if there were switching of excitation from one point to another, can actually occur under certain conditions.

We have thus examined the conditions under which excitation which has arisen on one side can pass to the other, namely when the intensity of this excitation is high or when, at the time of its development, there is on the opposite side of the brain latent or declared excitation of not less intensity.

The intensity with which excitation irradiates is inconstant: it may change even in the course of one experimental day (it changes markedly and generally reaches zero with increase

TABLE 9. DIMINISHING IRRADIATION OF EXCITATION FROM LEFT TO RIGHT ON CONTINUED APPLICATION OF UNCONDITIONED STIMULATION ON THE LEFT SIDE. EXPERIMENT ON THE DOG DEVONKA, 30 OCTOBER 1953.

Surface stimulated	Time of experiment	Unconditioned reflex salivation from parotid glands in each minute (scale divisions)	
		Left	Right
Left tongue segment	10·30 hr	360	90
	10·35 hr	440	50
	10·40 hr	460	35

in the number of applications of the corresponding stimulus). We know, for example, that if a tongue segment on either side is stimulated every 5 min with acid solution of the same strength, the salivary reaction on the side of stimulation increases gradually with each succeeding stimulation, and that the gland reaction declines gradually on the opposite side, the side to which the excitation irradiates. Details of an experiment are given to illustrate this (Table 9).

Further study of this problem (experiments of T. E. Kolosova) established that salivary secretion from the gland on the side opposite to that of the segment stimulated declined when a stimulus of increasing intensity was used, as well as with an unconditioned stimulus of the same intensity (the intensity of the stimulus was increased either by increasing the strength of the acid with which the tongue was painted or by increasing the number of times the tongue was painted with acid of the same strength).

TABLE 10. DIMINISHING IRRADIATION OF EXCITATION FROM RIGHT TO LEFT ON SUCCESSIVE INCREASE IN THE STRENGTH OF THE UNCONDITIONED STIMULATION ON THE RIGHT SIDE. EXPERIMENT ON THE DOG DEVONKA, 29 JANUARY 1958.

Surface stimulated	Unconditioned reflex salivation from parotid glands in each minute (scale divisions)	
	Left	Right
Right tongue segment (3 times)	40	110
Right tongue segment (6 times)	30	170
Right tongue segment (9 times)	0	240
Right tongue segment (12 times)	0	240

Table 10 shows that salivation from the gland on the side of stimulation (right) increased with each succeeding stimulation whereas salivary secretion from the left salivary gland declined and reached zero after the second stimulation.

Decline of salivation from the gland on the side opposite to stimulation, on the side of irradiation, was thus equally definite whether a stimulus of the same intensity or a stimulus of successively increased intensity was used. This decline of salivation is apparently the result of concentration of the excitation. The excitation which developed in one hemisphere passed to the opposite side and then returned gradually to its place of origin. In other words, the excitation irradiated initially but later became progressively more concentrated with each succeeding application of the stimulus. Parallel with this, irradiation diminished and finally disappeared completely, the excitation becoming concentrated on one side—the side of its initial development.

The basis of the mechanism for concentration of excitation is, as has long been known from conditioned reflex work, negative induction. It is thought that excitation develops in some focus in the central nervous system and then irradiates peripherally from this focus. At the same time there is at the periphery development of an induced inhibitory process—negative induction, which presents a counter-wave, turns the excitation back to the place of its development and concentrates it there. The gradual decline of salivation to zero on the side opposite to that stimulated should, therefore, be the result of negative induction.

It must, however, be assumed from the last experiments that the concentration of excitation is based on a more complex mechanism. Latent excitation would appear to be an important factor, as well as negative induction, in the process of excitation concentration. The basis for this assumption is the fact of which we spoke earlier. We saw in the preceding experiments that, when latent excitation developed, it attracted to itself a wave of declared excitation. The declared excitation thus began to be concentrated in the focus of latent excitation and this limited its irradiation partly or completely.

It was also established by our earlier experiments that the more powerful the action of the stimulus and the more powerful the declared excitation the more intense was the latent excitation which developed after it in its focus and the more powerfully it attracted any declared excitation to its own focus of origin. This fact reveals clearly a property of latent excitation which is diametrically the opposite to that of declared excitation. The stronger it is, the more and the more intensely does the latter irradiate. Latent excitation, on the other hand, attracts declared excitation to its own focus of origin and concentrates it there with increasing intensity as its own strength increases. On this evidence it must be recognized that one of the reasons for the concentration of powerful declared excitation is the associated development of a process of latent excitation. When the same stimulation is applied successively at regular intervals, each succeeding stimulation will have a greater effect than the preceding. The explanation is that, when applied the second time, the stimulus does not act alone but is supplemented by the latent excitation remaining after the first stimulation. Their summated action gives a greater effect and this in turn determines the development of more intense latent excitation than after the first stimulation. This more powerful excitation will attract the next stimulation more powerfully to the place of its own development and so restrict the irradiation of the succeeding excitation more powerfully, and so on. Consequently, with each succeeding application of the same stimulus, latent excitation in the focus for the stimulus in the central nervous system will increase gradually and, parallel with this, the intensity of the irradiation of the declared excitation will diminish gradually until finally it ceases altogether.

Reflex Arc for the Unilateral Unconditioned Salivary Reflex

When we speak of unilateral unconditioned salivary reflexes, we describe it as unilateral solely on the basis of the external effect—salivation, on the fact that, when a tongue segment on one side was stimulated, salivation developed on one side—

F

the side of stimulation. It does not, of course, follow from this that the central apparatus for unconditioned salivation is in one hemisphere. For example, if there is unconditioned salivation from the left salivary gland, this does not mean that, when a unilateral unconditioned stimulus is applied, the focus of excitation in the central nervous system is also on the left side; it may be on the right side or it may be on both sides.

Work to settle this question proceeded along two lines: it was essential, first, to determine the side on which the cortical part of the reflex arc for unconditioned salivation from the salivary gland on one side was situated and, secondly, to discover the place of origin in the central nervous system of the nerve fibres in this arc. Experiments were carried out on dogs by the old, well-tested and still valid method of extirpation.

TABLE 11. CHANGES IN PAROTID SALIVATION AFTER REMOVAL OF THE CORTEX OF THE RIGHT HEMISPHERE. EXPERIMENTS ON THE DOG GROM, OPERATION 10 JUNE 1952.

Salivation (ml) associated with the eating of 10 g meat-biscuit powder			
Before operation (17 May '52)		After operation (20 June '52)	
Left gland	Right gland	Left gland	Right gland
0·8	0·3	1·0	0·1
0·8	0·7	0·8	0·4
0·7	1·0	0·7	0·6
0·07	0·07	0·07	0·15
1·10	0·8	0·8	0·4
Total 4·0	2·87	3·37	1·65

In an attempt to settle the first question we determined the background unconditioned salivation in relation to the eating of a definite quantity of meat-biscuit powder, salivation being recorded for the parotid glands separately. This done, we removed the cortex of one hemisphere (for the manner of removal see Method) and, when the dog had recovered, we examined salivary secretion under the same conditions as before operation to determine what changes had occurred. Many such experiments were carried out and in all cases without exception we observed the same phenomenon: after unilateral decortication the value of the unconditioned salivary reflex was reduced on the same side, whereas the reflexes on the opposite side from the symmetrical salivary glands had their original values and retained them unchanged from the second postoperative day onwards; in a few cases the values were increased during the first few days after the operation.

TABLE 12. CHANGES IN PAROTID SALIVATION AFTER REMOVAL OF THE CORTEX OF THE RIGHT HEMISPHERE. EXPERIMENTS ON THE DOG MOLNIYA, OPERATION 2 OCTOBER 1952.

Salivation (scale divisions) associated with the eating of 10 g meat-biscuit powder			
Before operation (1 Oct. '52)		After operation (6 Oct. '52)	
Left gland	Right gland	Left gland	Right gland
1150	810	1020	185
1150	1100	940	156
1030	920	1235	165
1130	930	830	121
1190	1100	755	170
Total 5650	4860	4780	797

We describe the experiments on four dogs (Tables 11, 12, 13 and 14). All these experiments were carried out in the same way: the dog was given a certain quantity of moistened meat-biscuit powder (10 g) to eat, 5 times at intervals of 4 min on an experimental day; salivation was measured during the first 2 min after eating commenced by means of a graduated test tube or glass tubes (for each parotid gland separately). The dog took 60–80 sec to eat the meat-biscuit powder. The values of salivation for each successive feed and for the entire experimental day are given in the records.

It can be concluded from this group of experiments that the

TABLE 13. CHANGES IN PAROTID SALIVATION AFTER REMOVAL OF THE
LEFT HEMISPHERE. EXPERIMENTS ON THE DOG TUCHA, OPERATION
3 JANUARY 1953.

Salivation (ml) associated with eating of 10 g meat-biscuit powder

Before operation (3 Jan. '53)		After operation (13 Jan. '53)	
Left gland	Right gland	Left gland	Right gland
0·4	0·9	Traces	0·9
1·0	1·2	0·1	1·2
0·9	0·8	0·1	0·9
0·7	0·8	0·1	0·7
0·7	0·7	0·6	0·6
Total 3·7	4·4	1·0	4·3

TABLE 14. CHANGES IN PAROTID SALIVATION AFTER REMOVAL OF THE
CORTEX OF THE LEFT HEMISPHERE. EXPERIMENTS ON THE DOG GROZA,
OPERATION 24 JUNE 1952.

Salivation (ml) associated with eating of 10 g meat-biscuit powder

Before operation 24 June '52		After operation			
		30 June '52		9 July '52	
Left gland	Right gland	Left gland	Right gland	Left gland	Right gland
0·4	0·3	0·1	0·2	0·1	0·1
0·4	0·4	0·1	0·7	0·2	0·3
0·4	0·2	0·2	0·6	0·3	0·6
0·4	0·3	0·1	0·7	0·3	0·6
0·5	0·4	0·6	0·5	0·1	0·2
Total 2·1	1·6	1·1	2·7	1·0	1·8

cortical part of the reflex arc for the unconditioned reflex of
the salivary gland on one side is on the same side as the gland.
This suggested that the conducting paths for the un-

conditioned reflex arc might also be found on the same side.

We could not, however, fail to give consideration to long established anatomical findings that the ascending paths of the taste nerve crossed in the medulla. This would mean that, after unilateral decortication, the unconditioned salivary reflex would be reduced on the opposite side, and not on the side of decortication, which is not the result that we obtained in our experiments. In order to reconcile our results with the anatomical data, it was suggested that there was a second decussation of the ascending paths for the unconditioned salivary reflex.

If such a double decussation existed, the ascending paths starting from the receptive surface of the tongue segment on one side should cross a second time into the cortical part of the hemisphere on the side of the tongue segment and salivary glands. In order to determine the position of this decussation of the taste nerve we turned first of all to that important brain structure, the diencephalon; if it were assumed that the position of the second decussation of the taste nerve was in the optic thalamus, then it could be expected that removal of the optic thalamus on one side would produce a change in the unconditioned salivation of the gland on the opposite side.

We thus had to effect surgical removal of the optic thalamus and this we decided to tackle through the posterior part of the suprasylvian convolution and the hippocampus (see Method for removal of the optic thalamus). It was essential, before carrying out this operation, to determine the importance in relation to unconditioned salivation of those parts of the brain which would be removed to give access to the optic thalamus on one side. In preliminary experiments we established the level of unconditioned salivation from the salivary glands of each side in relation to the eating of meat-biscuit powder. We then removed the posterior part of the suprasylvian gyrus and the subjacent white substance down to the hippocampus which curves round behind the optic thalamus. Most of the pulvinar was thus exposed from behind and free access to the optic thalamus obtained. The wound was then sutured. The dogs tolerated this operation very well and were taken for experiment on the 2nd or 3rd postoperative day. Below we give details of an experiment with unconditioned salivary reflexes on one of the experimental dogs before and after the operation (Table 15).

TABLE 15. CHANGES IN PAROTID SALIVATION AFTER REMOVAL OF THE POSTERIOR PART OF THE SUPRASYLVIAN GYRUS AND THE HIPPOCAMPUS ON THE LEFT SIDE. EXPERIMENTS ON THE DOG ZOR'KA. OPERATION— 26 JULY 1955.

Salivation (ml) associated with eating of 10 g meat-biscuit powder			
Before operation (26 July '55)		After operation (29 July '55)	
Left gland	Right gland	Left gland	Right gland
0·4	0·4	0·3	0·5
0·7	0·6	0·7	1·1
0·9	0·9	0·5	0·8
0·5	0·6	1·0	0·5
0·5	0·5	0·5	0·3
Total 3·0	3·0	3·0	3·2

In order to establish the background unconditioned salivation, the dogs were given 10 g meat-biscuit powder 5 times at intervals of 4 min on one experimental day. Salivation was recorded over a period of 2 min from the time eating commenced for each parotid gland separately.

Table 15 shows that removal of these parts of the brain produced no changes in unconditioned salivation on the side of removal or on the opposite side.

On the evidence afforded by this experiment we could thus ascribe all the changes in unconditioned salivation associated with removal of the optic thalamus and damage to the part of the brain in the route thereto, to the removal of the optic thalamus.

In the experiments to establish the effect of removal of the optic thalamus the dog was prepared as in the preceding experiments (background unconditioned salivation was established and the optic thalamus was then removed). We give details of the experiments on two dogs (Tables 16 and 17).

TABLE 16. CHANGES IN PAROTID SALIVATION AFTER REMOVAL OF THE
LEFT OPTIC THALAMUS. EXPERIMENTS ON THE DOG CHERNOMOR.
OPERATION—10 JANUARY 1956.

Salivation (ml) associated with the eating of 10 g meat-biscuit powder

Before operation (31 Dec. '55)		After operation (19 Jan. '56)	
Left gland	Right gland	Left gland	Right gland
0·6	0·4	0·1	0·4
0·8	0·7	0·4	0·8
0·6	0·9	0·5	0·8
0·7	0·5	0·5	0·6
0·8	0·5	0·3	0·6
Total 3·5	3·0	1·8	3·2

TABLE 17. CHANGES IN PAROTID SECRETION AFTER REMOVAL OF THE
LEFT OPTIC THALAMUS. EXPERIMENTS ON THE DOG CHARODEI.
OPERATION—13 OCTOBER 1955.

Salivation (ml) associated with the eating of 10 g meat-biscuit powder

Before operation (13 Oct. '55)		After operation (26 Oct. '55)	
Left gland	Right gland	Left gland	Right gland
0·4	0·8	Traces	0·6
0·5	0·5	0·3	0·6
0·7	0·6	0·2	0·8
0·4	0·4	0·1	0·5
0·5	0·7	0·4	0·5
Total 2·5	3·0	1·0	3·0

These experiments showed that removal of one optic thalamus
led to reduction of the unconditioned reflexes on the side of
removal, whereas reflexes were unchanged on the opposite
side, the conclusion being that the ascending fibres of the
taste analyser did not cross in the optic thalamus.

We then established background unconditioned salivation in other dogs and transected one cerebral peduncle at the junction between the medial geniculate body and the anterior corpus quadrigeminum of the same side. We reproduce the experiments on two dogs (Tables 18 and 19).

TABLE 18.   CHANGE IN PAROTID SALIVATION AFTER DIVISION OF THE RIGHT CEREBRAL PEDUNCLE. EXPERIMENTS ON THE DOG KHRABRAYA. OPERATION—10 MARCH 1954.

Salivation (ml) associated with the eating of 10 g meat-biscuit powder

Before operation (2 March '54)		After operation (20 May '54)	
Left gland	Right gland	Left gland	Right gland
0·3	0·2	0·2	Traces
0·3	0·8	0·7	0·2
0·5	1·0	0·6	0·2
0·6	0·5	0·4	0·3
0·4	0·2	0·4	0·4
Total 2·1	2·7	2·3	1·1

TABLE 19.   CHANGES IN PAROTID SALIVATION AFTER DIVISION OF THE LEFT CEREBRAL PEDUNCLE. EXPERIMENTS ON THE DOG SMEL'CHAK. OPERATION—29 MARCH 1958.

Salivation (ml) associated with the eating of 10 g meat-biscuit powder

Before operation (27 May '58)		After operation (19 June '58)	
Left gland	Right gland	Left gland	Right gland
0·8	1·0	0·3	1·6
0·8	1·0	0·3	1·6
1·6	1·1	0·6	1·2
1·1	1·4	0·6	1·2
1·0	1·3	0·5	0·8
0·9	1·0	0·6	1·0
Total 5·4	5·8	2·6	5·8

In these experiments unconditioned salivation was reduced only on the side of operation. The next form of operation undertaken in an attempt to find an answer to our problem was transection of a lateral half of the medulla at the level of the middle angle of the rhomboid fossa (Table 20).

TABLE 20. CHANGES IN PAROTID SECRETION AFTER TRANSECTION OF THE RIGHT HALF OF THE MEDULLA. EXPERIMENTS ON THE DOG BUYAN. OPERATION—15 JULY 1954.

Before operation (11 June '54)		After operation (2 Aug. '54)	
Left gland	Right gland	Left gland	Right gland
0·9	0·7	0·7	0·1
1·2	1·3	1·2	0·5
1·0	0·8	1·1	0·4
0·8	0·8	0·9	0·5
0·5	0·3	0·8	0·2
Total 4·4	3·9	4·7	1·7

Salivation from parotid glands (ml) associated with the eating of 10 g meat-biscuit powder

With this as with the preceding operations, the unconditioned reflexes were reduced on the side of operation and those on the opposite side were unchanged.

Another operation carried out on fresh dogs was removal of the caudate body on one side (see Method, Chapter I). There was no change in unconditioned salivation on either side after these operations.

Our investigation thus demonstrated that there was no second crossing of the taste nerve anywhere in the nerve formations of the brain. It then became quite clear that the excitation originating from stimulation of the receptive surface of a tongue segment on one side entered the cortex of the same side, having travelled, contrary to published data, over a direct path on the same side.

These experiments enabled us to correct our earlier theory:

G

solely on the basis of published data (Rauber, 1911; Bekhterev, 1896), and not having the evidence afforded by extirpation of different parts of the brain, we had suggested that the ascending and descending fibres of the taste analyser crossed to the opposite side (Abuladze, 1953). This view has not been confirmed by our experiments and it must be regarded as quite evident that, when a tongue segment on any one side is stimulated, the excitation travels over nerve paths and develops in a part of the central formations which lie on the same side as the stimulated tongue segment and the salivary glands.

As was seen earlier, unconditioned stimulation of a tongue segment on one side led to reaction, exclusively or mainly, by the salivary gland on that side. Unilateral unconditioned stimulation never led to identical reactions by the two glands, either in time or intensity.

When a weak unconditioned stimulus acted on one side, only one gland reacted and the other gland remained quiescent; when an unconditioned stimulus of one intensity acted on one side and another stimulus of a different intensity acted on the other, there was a corresponding difference in the intensity of salivation from the glands. The paired salivary glands can be made to function separately just like paired motor organs (extremities).

There is then the question of whether, on analogy with these symmetrical organs, which can clearly be made to function separately, symmetrical parts of the cerebral cortex, the anatomical structure of which is bilaterally symmetrical, can be brought into activity separately. This question of the separate functioning of the cortices of the two hemispheres is difficult and complex. In Pavlov's expression, the cortex is the organ of higher nervous activity, and we are accustomed to think of it as functioning as a single integral organ, as a single integral formation. For example, no one has ever been able to say on which side of the brain or, more correctly, in which hemisphere nervous processes are occurring at a particular moment. No one can sense on which side of the brain mental activity is proceeding at a particular moment. Consequently, the question of any such disjunction or dissociation of functioning in the cortex is not acute or does not, in fact, arise. It should, however, be emphasized that definite evidence has been accumulating recently, from which it can be concluded that the view on possible separate functioning of symmetrical parts of the cerebral cortex is perfectly legitimate.

Unilateral Salivary Conditioned Reflexes

The classical method for the formation of salivary conditioned reflexes in dogs is, of course, the combination of indifferent stimuli with the eating of meat-biscuit powder, that is the combination of an indifferent stimulus with stimulation of the entire mouth cavity. We effected some modification of this method for the formation of conditioned reflexes for the particular problem we were investigating. The change was that the action of an indifferent stimulus was combined with stimulation of the mucous membrane on exteriorized symmetrical segments of the posterior third of the tongue, and not with stimulation of the entire mouth cavity. As we have already noted, separate stimulation of each segment elicited salivation mainly or exclusively (depending on the strength of the stimulus) on the side of stimulation only. When the action of an indifferent stimulus was combined with unconditioned stimulation of the mucosa of an exteriorized tongue segment, a "unilateral conditioned reflex" was formed. Four forms of unconditioned stimulation of the mucosa of the two exteriorized tongue segments were used.

(1) Weak unconditioned stimulation of one side elicited salivation on one side only. When an indifferent stimulus was combined with a weak unconditioned stimulus a conditioned reflex was elaborated on one side only, the side of action of the unconditioned stimulus.

(2) Strong unconditioned stimulation of one side elicited salivation from both glands, but more on the side of stimulation and much less on the opposite side. When an indifferent stimulus was combined with a powerful unconditioned stimulus, a conditioned reflex was still formed on one side only (the side of action of the unconditioned stimulus). This phenomenon is

one that has long attracted our attention, even in the very early experiments with unilateral conditioned reflexes, and was somewhat unexpected.

A new form of application of the unconditioned stimulation (3) was tried in an effort to explain the production of this phenomenon.

(3) This form of unconditioned stimulation was the simultaneous action on the exteriorized tongue segments of two unconditioned stimuli of different intensities (Lapina, 1954). In these experiments the left tongue segment was stimulated with a strong acid solution (HCl 0·33 N) and the right segment was stimulated with a weak acid solution (HCl 0·1 N). Unconditioned salivation was correspondingly greater on the left than on the right side. The metronome 120/min was combined with this pair of unconditioned reflexes.

Experiments of this nature established that a conditioned reflex was formed on the side of action of the strong unconditioned reflex, the side of more intense salivation—in our case the left side. When the powerful unconditioned reflex on the left side was excluded from this pair of unconditioned reflexes, a reflex to the same metronome then appeared on the right side, to disappear again on that side and reappear on the left side with restoration of the action of the original pair of unconditioned reflexes. This example shows that when an indifferent stimulus was combined with two unconditioned stimuli of different strengths acting on tongue segments on the respective sides, the powerful unconditioned stimulus interferes in some way with the formation and development of a conditioned reflex on the side of the weak unconditioned stimulus.

(4) In the fourth form of unconditioned stimulation the two stimuli act simultaneously and with the same intensity on the receptive surfaces on both sides. In this case a conditioned reflex is always formed simultaneously on both right and left. An example of the formation of such a conditioned reflex is afforded by the classical experiments with alimentary conditioned reflexes in which an indifferent stimulus is combined with the eating of meat-biscuit powder. In such an experimental arrangement the conditioned stimulus is combined with

identical unconditioned stimulation of the mouth cavity on both sides.

The forms in which an indifferent stimulus was combined with the unconditioned stimulation of the symmetrical, exteriorized tongue segments also varied. We know that the receptive surfaces for the analysers (visual, auditory and cutaneous) are paired and symmetrical. Consequently, when conditioned reflexes are elaborated by combinations of stimulation of these analysers with stimulation of the exteriorized tongue segments, both analyser and mucous membrane of the tongue segment being stimulated separately, there are nine forms in which the conditioned and unconditioned stimuli can be combined (Table 21).

TABLE 21.   VARIOUS COMBINATIONS OF UNILATERAL CONDITIONED
AND UNCONDITIONED STIMULI.

Combination	Side of conditioned stimulation	Side of unconditioned stimulation
1st form	Left	Left
2nd ,,	Left	Right
3rd ,,	Right	Right
4th ,,	Right	Left
5th ,,	Left	Left and Right
6th ,,	Right	Left and Right
7th ,,	Left and Right	Left
8th ,,	Left and Right	Right
9th ,,	Left and Right	Left and Right

The classical method of elaborating salivary conditioned reflexes on the basis of the unconditioned alimentary reflex, that is on the basis of stimulation of the entire receptive surface in the mouth cavity, corresponds to the 5th, 6th and 9th forms in the scheme of combinations.

In the 1st form the combination "left–left" means that both stimuli, conditioned and unconditioned, acted on the corresponding peripheral receptive surface on the left side. If we consider the sides of action of the combined stimulations at the time when they are acting on the cortical region, a schema of the sides of their influences would not be the same as the schema given, as the ascending paths of many analysers cross. If a visual conditioned stimulus of one side, say the left eye, is combined with stimulation of the left tongue segment, then at the periphery the combined conditioned and unconditioned stimuli will act on one side, namely the left, and the form of the combination will be unilateral, "left–left", but it will not be unilateral in the central region and the form of combination will be "right–left". This is due to the fact that the ascending paths of the visual system in the dog are crossed so that stimulation of the left eye creates excitation in the right hemisphere. The importance of coincidence or non-coincidence of the sides of action of combined stimuli will be discussed later when we examine the location of the conditioned reflex arc for salivation.

It should be noted that the side on which a salivary conditioned reflex is formed is determined by the side of action of the unconditioned stimulus, and not that of the conditioned stimulus. In whichever form of the above schema or in whatever intensity or quantity the conditioned stimulus is combined with the unconditioned, the conditioned reflex is invariably, right from the moment of its first appearance, elaborated on the side of action of the unconditioned stimulus. This is the pattern observed: if the unconditioned salivary reflex is unilateral, the conditioned reflex is also elaborated on that side; if the unconditioned reflex is bilateral and of different intensities, the conditioned reflex becomes attached to the side of the strong unconditioned reflex; and finally, the conditioned reflex is elaborated on both sides if the unconditioned reflex is bilateral and of uniform intensity.

These experiments showed that it was easy to elaborate in the same dog a salivary conditioned reflex to one or to several stimuli on one side and a conditioned reflex to a series of other independent stimuli on the other side.

We give details of two reflexes in the same dog by way of illustration (Tables 22 and 23).

It is quite obvious that conditioned excitation, like other forms of excitation examined earlier (unconditioned, latent), can develop and be maintained on one side. But conditioned

TABLE 22. RIGHT-SIDED CONDITIONED REFLEX. EXPERIMENT ON THE
DOG ANTARES, 24 JULY 1951.

Time of experiment	Stimulus	No. of combi-nation	Parotid salivation (scale divisions)			
			Left gland		Right gland	
			Cond.	Uncond.	Cond.	Uncond.
11.55 hr	M–120	366	0	58	10	190
12.00 hr	M–120	367	0	30	15	190

NOTE: Metronome was reinforced on right side.

TABLE 23. LEFT-SIDED CONDITIONED REFLEX. EXPERIMENT ON DOG
ANTARES, 25 JULY 1951.

Time of experiment	Stimulus	No. of combi-nation	Parotid salivation (scale divisions)			
			Left gland		Right gland	
			Cond.	Uncond.	Cond.	Uncond.
11.58 hr	Bell	316	15	215	0	45
12.03 hr	Bell	317	12	189	0	0

excitation which has developed in one hemisphere can also pass to the opposite side under certain conditions. One of the main conditions for this is the presence of latent excitation on the opposite side.

The following illustrates this. When the beating of a metronome was combined with stimulation of the left tongue segment, a unilateral conditioned reflex was elaborated after a certain time, which meant that the metronome would elicit a conditioned reaction in the salivary glands of the left side only and that the right salivary gland would not react to the metronome. The experiment was carried out in the way shown in Table 24 on one experimental day.

It is quite obvious that the excitation associated with the

TABLE 24. "DISPLACEMENT" OF A LEFT-SIDED CONDITIONED REFLEX
TO THE RIGHT SIDE AFTER PRIOR EXCITATION OF THE RIGHT SALIVARY
GLAND. EXPERIMENT ON THE DOG DEVONKA, 20 DECEMBER 1959.

Time	Stimulus	No. of com-bina-tion	Parotid salivation (scale divisions)		Salivation on painting of right tongue segment with 0·1 N HCl for 2 sec (secretion in each 10-sec period)
			Left gland	Right gland	
11.55 hr	M–120	130	20	0	
12.00 hr	M–120	131	30	0	
12.10 hr	—	—	—	–	60
					50
					30
					10
					0
12.15 hr	M–120	132	0	20	

metronome deviated completely from the elaborated path and
went to the salivary gland of the right, and not the left side,
that is, it was directed to the side on which latent excitation
had previously been created. When the conditioned stimulus,
the metronome, was applied a second time or at a longer
interval (10–20 min) after the end of the preliminary salivation
on the right side, when the latent excitation had already
disappeared there, the metronome elicited its own conditioned
reflex on its own side.

A salivary conditioned reflex elaborated on one side can be
freed from the influence of latent excitation on the opposite
side by prolonged "training". The metronome has to be
contraposed to the latent excitation a great many times before
the metronome, applied after a fairly short interval (5 min)
ultimately produces a conditioned reflex on its own side. When
attained, however, this position is relatively unstable, and the
conditioned excitation from the metronome deviates from its
own path and goes to the side of latent excitation if work with

the metronome is interrupted or if the intensity of the unconditioned stimulus is altered.

If latent excitation is produced by a weak conditioned
stimulus or if the conditioned stimulus is applied long after the
development of the latent excitation, when the latter is already
beginning to decline, the conditioned reflex to the metronome
is split: it appears partly on its own side and partly on the
opposite side.

There are two possible explanations for the deviation of the
path of the conditioned excitation. (1) When salivation ceases,
latent excitation develops on the right side and this "attracts"
the conditioned excitation from the metronome applied
immediately thereafter. (2) It is conceivable that the application of the unconditioned stimulus on the right side produces
negative induction on the opposite left side and the conditioned
stimulus on the left side fails to act as a result of this negative
induction.

Such an explanation immediately raises the question of the
part of the central nervous system on the left side (on which the
conditioned reflex was elaborated) in which the negative
induction causing the inhibition which prevents the development of a conditioned effect on that side develops—whether
at the point of action of the conditioned stimulus or at the
point of action of the unconditioned stimulus reinforcing it.
It is clear that there is no negative induction at the point in the
central nervous system corresponding to the conditioned
stimulation. The conditioned stimulus produces a large positive
effect, admittedly not on its own side but on the opposite side,
but it nevertheless produces such an effect. This indicates
that the point corresponding to the conditioned stimulus in the
cortex is not inhibited. Consequently, the absence of a conditioned reflex on the side of the conditioned stimulus—the left
side—after preliminary excitation of the right side is difficult
to explain by the presence of negative induction in the point
of application of the conditioned stimulus. Neither can it be
thought that the negative induction which developed after
application of the unconditioned stimulus to the right side in
our experiments was in the central nervous system on the left

H

side at the point corresponding to the left-sided unconditioned stimulus.

This conclusion had been arrived at on the evidence provided by numerous experiments in our earlier investigations on unilateral unconditioned salivary reflexes. The following was constantly observed in these investigations: if the unconditioned stimulus was applied on one side, say the right, and if, when salivation on that side had ceased, stimulation was applied to the tongue segment on the opposite (left) side, on which there should presumably be negative induction, the unconditioned stimulus produced the usual reflex on the left side and much irradiation on the opposite, right side. This fact showed that no inhibition produced by the mechanism of negative induction could be demonstrated on the left side and that consequently, the point of application of the unconditioned stimulus in the central nervous system on the left side was not inhibited, that is, was not under the influence of negative induction produced by the preliminary stimulation of the opposite right side.

The more probable of the two explanations offered for this phenomenon is, therefore, that the prior application of the unconditioned stimulus on the right side led to the development of latent excitation which attracted the conditioned excitation to its own side. The result was that the conditioned stimulus produced a positive effect, not on its own side but on the side of latent excitation, the side on which the unconditioned stimulus had previously acted.

The fact that any declared excitation (conditioned or unconditioned) deviates towards a focus of latent excitation enables us to state with a considerable degree of probability that latent excitation is one of the important components in the mechanism for the formation of the ordinary salivary conditioned reflex. When, for the formation of a conditioned reflex, an indifferent stimulus is reinforced by an unconditioned stimulus, every time it acts, latent excitation is left behind in the same place in the central nervous system after its action. This persists until the next application of the indifferent stimulus, the excitation from which is invariably directed to the side of the focus for the unconditioned stimulus.

Thus, the first factor directing the excitation from the conditioned stimulus to the unconditioned is latent excitation. The unconditioned reinforcement which follows this can only favour the strengthening of this connection and develop the paths from the point of conditioned to that of unconditioned excitation.

Further experiments showed that inhibition as well as excitation could develop and be maintained on one side. Positive salivary conditioned reflexes were elaborated separately to three stimuli in the experiments of Travina (1952b). One of these stimuli was reinforced by an unconditioned salivary reflex on one side and two separate reflexes by an unconditioned salivary reflex of the other side. When the background values of the conditioned reflexes to the several stimuli had been established, the two stimuli were applied simultaneously on one side on one of the experimental days. When the experiment was carried out in this way, not only was the total effect less than the sum of the values of the conditioned reflexes to each of the stimuli separately but it was less than each of those values. This phenomenon was explained by the intervention of prohibitive inhibition. The strength of the two stimuli applied simultaneously on the one side apparently exceeded the functional capacity of the central nervous system on this side with the result that there was development of prohibitive inhibition and the reflexes were reduced.

The important point here was that the prohibitive inhibition was only on the stimulated side. This was easily proved if, soon after cessation of the simultaneous action of the two stimuli on the one side with reduced effect, the conditioned stimulus for the opposite side was applied; it produced a reflex of the usual value and no effect of the prohibitive inhibition could be observed. This shows that there was prohibitive inhibition, fatigue, loss of functional capacity on the one side and full functional capacity on the opposite side.

The experiments of M. M. Khananashvili, who happened to use in his work a dog with, right from the start, reduced functional capacity on one side of the central nervous system, were consistent with these findings. Unilateral conditioned reflexes to acoustic and cutaneous stimulations were elaborated in this dog. The reflexes were elaborated equally quickly on both the right and left sides and rapidly reached constant and almost identical values. It was found on further work, however, that the reflexes on one side to all the stimuli began to decline steadily, finally reaching zero, whereas the conditioned reflexes of the opposite side remained unchanged. The conditioned stimuli were changed several times in the case of this dog but the results were always the same; the reflexes to any new stimuli were elaborated equally well on both sides. After several weeks of further work, however, the conditioned reflexes began to decline to zero always on the same side and the conditioned reflexes on the opposite side remained unchanged. There is no other explanation for this phenomenon than functional defect of the one hemisphere. The reason for this reduced functional capacity in one hemisphere was not quite clear, but it persisted throughout the entire period of work with the dog—about three years.

Conditioned inhibition can also develop and be maintained unilaterally. Lapina (1956a, 1956b) elaborated unilateral salivary conditioned reflexes, one lot of conditioned stimuli being addressed to one side and another lot to the opposite side. Conditioned inhibition was elaborated to one of the stimuli on one side in the usual manner. Application of the conditioned inhibitor is known to be followed by the development of successive inhibition, particularly during the early period of work with it. It was found in Lapina's experiments that application of the conditioned inhibitor was followed by successive inhibition of the conditioned reflexes on the side of the conditioned inhibitor and that the conditioned reflexes on the opposite side were quite unchanged.

The same position was seen to develop in experiments with extinction. When we extinguished a conditioned reflex on one side, there was successive inhibition of the reflexes to stimuli which acted on the side of extinction and the conditioned reflexes on the opposite side remained unchanged.

It follows from these experiments that the forms of inhibition indicated (prohibitive, conditioned and extinctive) can develop and be maintained on one side without affecting the opposite side. The inhibitory process is retained on one side under certain conditions but, under other conditions, inhibition which develops on one side can also pass to the opposite side. Only one of all the conditions which can determine transfer of inhibition from one side to the other has so far been investigated by us, and that not completely. This condition is change in the intensity of the inhibition. Inhibition can remain on one side and reduce the effects of action of positive stimuli only on its own side so long as it does not exceed a certain medium intensity. If inhibition begins to deepen and its intensity to increase, it then passes to the opposite side as well and gradually reduces the effects of positive conditioned stimuli on this side in addition to reducing the effects of the positive stimuli on its own side.

Reflex Arc of the Salivary Conditioned Reflex

We stated earlier, when discussing the experiments with unconditioned salivary reflexes, that the production of unilateral unconditioned salivary reflexes could in no way be regarded as implying that the processes in the central parts of the nervous system were also unilateral. This statement can also be made in relation to conditioned reflexes. If, for example, we have a salivary conditioned reflex on one side, it does not follow that the conditioned salivary reaction of the one gland is effected by the cortex of one side only. It is conceivable that the cortex of both hemispheres may be involved in the production of a salivary conditioned reaction on one side. The method of extirpation was used on dogs to decide this problem, just as for determination of the side on which the cortical representation of the unconditioned salivary reflex was situated.

Below we give the results of experiments on two dogs mentioned by us earlier in connection with the investigation of unconditioned reflexes (Groza and Chernomor). These experiments illustrate the changes produced in conditioned reflexes by extirpation of the cortex and optic thalamus of one hemisphere.

An alimentary conditioned reflex to a bell was elaborated

in the dog Groza before removal of the cortex of the left hemisphere. This stimulus was combined with the eating of a certain quantity of meat-biscuit powder and the salivary reflexes, both conditioned and unconditioned, were recorded from the parotid gland on each side (Tables 25 and 26).

This dog had a left-sided acid reflex as well as the alimentary conditioned reflex. A metronome 120/min, acting alone for 20 sec, was combined with stimulation of the left tongue segment with decinormal hydrochloric acid. We give below the results of the experiments before and after removal of the cortex of the left hemisphere (Tables 27 and 28).

TABLE 25. ALIMENTARY CONDITIONED AND UNCONDITIONED REFLEXES IN BOTH PAROTID GLANDS. EXPERIMENT ON THE DOG GROZA, 23 JUNE 1952

Time	Stimulus	No. of combi- nation	Parotid salivation (scale units) before operation for removal of cortex			
			Left gland		Right gland	
			Cond.	Uncond.	Cond.	Uncond.
10.45 hr	Bell	52	13	297	20	215
10.50 hr	Bell	53	25	250	15	260
10.55 hr	Bell	54	22	290	25	260

These experiments (Tables 25 and 26) show that the alimentary conditioned reflex on the left side, the side of decortication, disappeared after removal of the left cortex and was not restored, even though the number of combinations of the conditioned stimulus (bell) with the eating of meat-biscuit powder after the operation reached 315 (the last combination before operation was No. 54 and after operation No. 369). The conditioned alimentary reflex to the same stimulus on the right side was unchanged: it developed constantly and had its original value. The left-sided acid conditioned reflex to M–120 (see Tables 27 and 28) likewise disappeared after removal of the cortex on the same side and was not restored although

TABLE 26. CHANGES IN THE VALUES OF CONDITIONED AND UNCONDITIONED PAROTID GLAND REFLEXES AFTER REMOVAL OF THE CORTEX OF THE LEFT HEMISPHERE. EXPERIMENT ON THE DOG GROZA, OPERATION 24 JUNE 1952.

Time	Stimulus	No. of combination	Parotid salivation (scale divisions)			
			Left gland		Right gland	
			Cond.	Uncond.	Cond.	Uncond.
Experiment of 8 Jan. '52						
01.05 hr	Bell	64	0	187	20	275
01.10 hr	Bell	65	0	155	10	190
01.15 hr	Bell	66	0	113	20	260
01.20 hr	Bell	67	0	149	25	280
Experiment of 6 Oct. '52						
12.14 hr	Bell	366	0	170	10	230
12.19 hr	Bell	367	0	150	15	260
12.24 hr	Bell	368	0	130	20	300
12.29 hr	Bell	369	0	160	15	205

TABLE 27. VALUES OF THE LEFT-SIDED ACID CONDITIONED AND UNCONDITIONED REFLEXES BEFORE REMOVAL OF THE CORTEX OF THE LEFT HEMISPHERE. EXPERIMENT ON THE DOG GROZA, 20 JUNE 1952.

Time	Stimulus	No. of combination	Parotid salivation (scale divisions)	
			Left gland	
			Conditioned	Unconditioned
10.45 hr	M–120	16	10	340
10.50 hr	M–120	17	10	375

the number of combinations reached 84 (17 before the operation, 101 after). At the same time, a right-sided unilateral reflex to a

TABLE 28. CHANGES IN THE VALUES OF THE LEFT-SIDED CONDITIONED AND UNCONDITIONED ACID REFLEXES AFTER REMOVAL OF THE CORTEX OF THE LEFT HEMISPHERE (THE OPERATION WAS CARRIED OUT ON 24 JUNE 1952). EXPERIMENT ON THE DOG GROZA, 10 JULY 1952.

Time	Stimulus	No. of combination	Salivation (scale divisions)	
			Left gland	
			Conditioned	Unconditioned
10.10 hr	M–120	100	0	230
10.15 hr	M–120	101	0	235

TABLE 29. RIGHT-SIDED ACID REFLEXES AFTER REMOVAL OF THE CORTEX OF THE LEFT HEMISPHERE. EXPERIMENTS ON THE DOG GROZA.

Time	Stimulus	No. of Combination	Parotid salivation (scale divisions)			
			Left gland		Right gland	
			Cond.	Uncond.	Cond.	Uncond.
Experiment of 18 Aug. '52						
11.17 hr	Whistle	16	–	–	12	245
11.22 hr	Whistle	17	–	–	20	250
Experiment of 22 Aug. '52						
11.31 hr	Whistle	21	–	–	10	240
11.36 hr	Whistle	22	–	–	15	245
Experiment of 27 Oct. '52						
10.32 hr	Whistle	50	–	–	20	385
10.37 hr	Whistle	51	–	–	15	375

whistle was elaborated rapidly. The whistle was combined with stimulation of the right tongue segment. The conditioned reflex on the right side was formed at the 16th combination and was constant thereafter. We give the results of three experiments at various periods (Table 29).

The bell was combined with the eating of meat-biscuit powder in experiments on this dog after almost five and a half years (9 July 1958). The bell was delivered simultaneously with food four or five times on an experimental day. After 30 such combinations the bell was made to act alone for 20 sec (Table 30). There had been 369 combinations before this long interval

TABLE 30. VALUES OF THE ALIMENTARY CONDITIONED AND UN-CONDITIONED REFLEXES IN BOTH PAROTID GLANDS (SCALE DIVISIONS) 5·5 YEARS AFTER REMOVAL OF THE CORTEX OF THE LEFT HEMISPHERE. EXPERIMENT ON THE DOG GROZA, 26 JULY 1958.

Time	Stimulus	No. of combination	Left gland		Right gland	
			Cond.	Uncond.	Cond.	Uncond.
13.05 hr	Bell	419	0	270	10	545
13.10 hr	Bell	420	0	205	10	535
13.15 hr	Bell	421	0	340	10	480
13.20 hr	Bell	422	0	228	15	570

and during this period after the operation no convulsive attacks of any kind were noted, the dog's general condition remained good and its weight remained steady. Despite this, the conditioned reflexes on the left side were not restored.

The optic thalamus was removed in the other dog Chernomor. This dog had no conditioned reflexes before the operation. The elaboration of a conditioned reflex was started on 20 January 1956. A whistle, acting alone for 20 sec, was combined with the eating of meat-biscuit powder. A conditioned reflex appeared on the right side after 10 combinations and became constant but the value of the reflex on the left side was zero and it remained at this level to the end of our experiments—the 115th combination (Table 31).

J

TABLE 31. VALUES OF THE ALIMENTARY CONDITIONED AND UN-
CONDITIONED REFLEXES IN THE PAROTID GLANDS AFTER REMOVAL OF
THE LEFT OPTIC THALAMUS. EXPERIMENT ON THE DOG CHERNOMOR,
17 FEBRUARY 1956.

Time	Stimulus	No. of combi- nation	Parotid salivation (scale divisions)			
			Left gland		Right gland	
			Cond.	Uncond.	Cond.	Uncond.
12.27 hr	Whistle	111	0	350	30	360
12.32 hr	Whistle	112	0	390	60	540
12.37 hr	Whistle	113	0	400	70	630
12.42 hr	Whistle	114	0	400	60	630
12.47 hr	Whistle	115	0	380	50	590

Experiments in which the cortex was removed unilaterally
showed clearly that this operation was followed by disappearance of salivary conditioned reflexes on the side of the removal
and that such reflexes could not thereafter be elaborated.
Conditioned reflexes on the opposite side remained unchanged.
These facts were quite definite and could be readily and
regularly demonstrated in all experiments without exception.
The only conclusion that could be arrived at from these experiments was that the removal of the cortex of one hemisphere
damaged the conditioned reflex arc for the salivary gland of one
side. But the disappearance of the conditioned reflex on one
side could not tell us whether the entire conditioned reflex arc
was destroyed or only part of it and, if the latter, then what
part. In the attempt to answer this question it had to be remembered that two analysers, those for the conditioned and unconditioned stimulations, were involved in the reflex arc for
the conditioned salivary reflex. The schema indicated earlier
(see Table 21) showed that the cortical parts of these analysers
were in one hemisphere (e.g. "left–left") in some cases and in
both hemispheres ("left–right") in others. Consequently, the
conditioned reflex always disappeared when the cortex of one
hemisphere was removed, but its disappearance depended

either on removal of the cortical parts of both analysers—conditioned and unconditioned—or on removal of one of them, either conditioned or unconditioned.

All the above experimental evidence relating to the functioning of the cerebral cortex in the dog enables us to underline three main properties of the cortex: the cerebral cortex functions on the principle of bilateral symmetry; under some conditions symmetrical parts may function separately while under other conditions the cortex functions as a single whole. The entire reflex arc of the unconditioned salivary reflex lies on one side, the side of the salivary gland and the receptive surface. The reflex arc for the conditioned salivary reflex is in one hemisphere in some cases and in both in others.

In discussing replacements of the function of removed or damaged parts of the cortex or of subjacent parts one must always start with recognition of the reflex arc as the essential substrate for any reaction. If the reflex arc is interrupted and there are no possible circuitous connections for its restoration, no reaction, conditioned or unconditioned, can be effected even though all the rest of the central nervous system and, in the case of man, his entire consciousness is in the most favourable state.

REFERENCES

ABULADZE, K. S. (1949) *The Summation Reflex. Research in Pavlov's Laboratory.* (Summatsionnyi refleks. Trudy laboratorii I. P. Pavlova.) Vol. 15.

ABULADZE, K. S. (1953) *A Study of Reflex Activity in Salivary and Lachrymal Glands* (Izucheniye reflektornoi deyatal'nosti slyunnykh i sleznykh zhelez).

BEKHTEREV, V. M. (1896) *Conducting Paths of the Spinal Cord and Brain* (Provodyashchiye puti spinnogo i golovnogo mozga).

ELLENBERGER, W. and BAUM, H. (1891) *Anatomie des Hundes.*

GAVRILOVA, L. N. (1954) *On the Functioning of Symmetrical Points in the Sensory Cortex (cutaneous analyser).* Proceedings of a Conference on the results of research in 1953, Institute of Experimental Medicine, U.S.S.R. Academy of Medical Sciences (K voprosu o funktsionirovanii dvukh simmetrichnykh punktov kozhnogo alalizatora. Tez. dokl. konf. po e itogam nauchno-issled. raboty za 1953 g.). Leningrad.

GAVRILOVA, L. N. (1959) *Effect of Unilateral Destruction of the Thalamus on the Course of Conditioned and Unconditioned Alimentary Reflexes.* Annual Report of the Institute of Experimental Medicine, U.S.S.R. Academy of Medical Sciences (Vliyaniye odnostoronnego razrusheniya talamusa na protekaniye uslovnykh i bezuslovnykh pishchevykh refleksov. Yezhegodnik IEM Akad. Med. Nauk SSSR). Vol. 4.

GAVRILOVA, L. N. (1960) Differentiation of symmetrical points on the skin in dogs by the side of action of an unconditioned stimulus. *Zh. vyssh. nervn. deyat.* **10**, 2.

GAVRILOVA, L. N. and TRAVINA, A. A. (1954) *The Summation of Residual with Immediate Excitation.* Proceedings of 3rd Conference of Junior Research Workers, Institute of Experimental Medicine, U.S.S.R. Academy of Medical Sciences. (Summatsiya ostatochnogo vozbuzhdeniya s nalichnym. Tez. dokl. III nauchn. konf. molodykh nauchn. rabotn., IEM Akad. Med. Nauk SSSR). Leningrad.

GAVRILOVA, L. N. and LAPINA, I. A. (1958) Period of persistence of residual excitation in the chemical (oral) analyser of the dog. *Zh. vyssh. nervn. deyat.* **8**, 3.

KOLOSOVA, T. Ye. (1959) *Irradiation and Concentration of the Excitatory Process Associated with Unilateral Stimulation of the Tongue.* Annual Report of the Institute of Experimental Medicine, Academy of Medical Sciences (Irradiatsiya i kontsentratsiya vozbuditel'nogo protsessa pri odnostoronnem razdrazhenii yazyka. Ezhegodnik IEM Akad. Med. Nauk SSSR). Leningrad.

LAPINA, I. A. (1953a) Irradiation in the salivary centre. *Fiziol. zh. SSSR* **39**, 3.

LAPINA, I. A. (1953b) *Relationship Between Symmetrical Salivation Centres.* Proceedings of a Scientific Conference of young research workers, Inst. Exp. Med., U.S.S.R. Acad. Med. Sciences (K voprosu o vzaimootnoshenii simmetrichnykh slyunootdelitel'nykh punktov. Tez. dokl. nauchn. konf. molodykh uchenykh, IEM Akad. Med. Nauk SSSR). Leningrad.

LAPINA, I. A. (1954) The formation of a conditioned salivary reflex on the basis of a compound unconditioned stimulus. *Fiziol. zh. SSSR* **40**, 6.

LAPINA, I. A. (1955) *The Cortical Representation of the Unconditioned Reflex.* Proceedings of 8th All-Union Congress of Physiologists, Biochemists and Pharmacologists (O korkovom predstavitel'stve bezuslovnogo refleksa. Trud. VIII Vses. s"exda fiziol., biokhim. i farmakol.), p. 716.

LAPINA, I. A. (1956a) Period of persistence of successive inhibition after extinction of unilateral reflexes. *Zh. vyssh. nervn. deyat.* **6**, 2.

LAPINA, I. A. (1956b) *The Differentiation of Acoustic Stimuli by the Side of Action.* Proceedings of 4th Conference of Junior Research Workers, Institute of Experimental Medicine, U.S.S.R. Academy of Medical Sciences (Differentsirovaniye zvukovykh razdrazhitelei, otlichayushchikhsya storonoi deistviya. Tez. IV konf. molodykh nauchn. rabotn. IEM Akad. Med. Nauk SSSR). Leningrad.

LAPINA, I. A. (1957) Residual (latent) excitation. *Byull. eksp. biol. i med.* **43**, 1.

LAPINA, I. A. (1958) Period of persistence of a focus of residual excitation in the chemical oral analyser of the dog. *Zh. vyssh. nervn. deyat.* **8**, 3.

RAUBER, A. (1911) *Handbook of Human Anatomy.* Vol. 5. Nervous system.

TRAVINA, A. A. (1952a) Conditioned reflexes based on stimulation of exteriorized tongue segments with food substances. *Zh. vyssh. nervn. deyat.* **2**, 1.

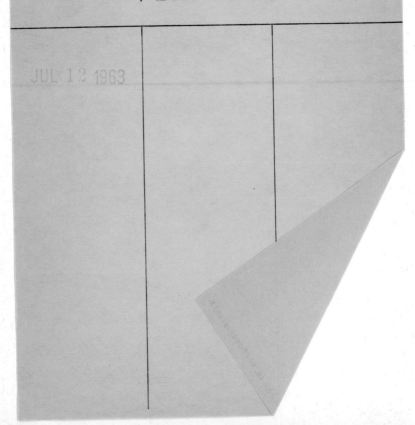